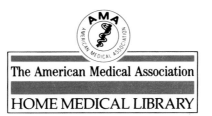

The American Medical Association

HOME MEDICAL LIBRARY

# WOMEN'S HEALTH

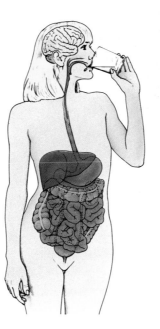

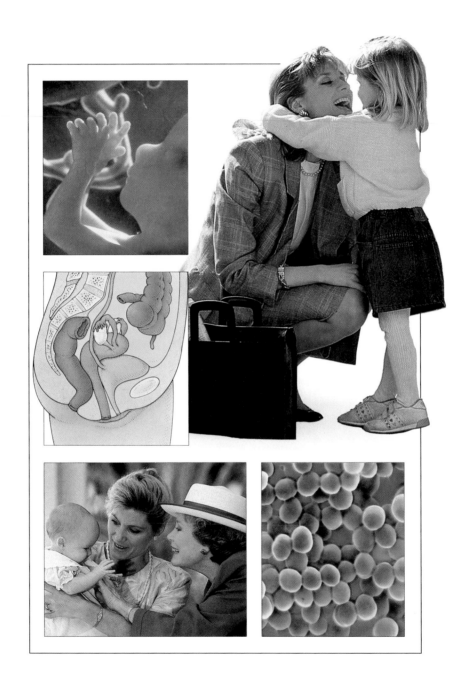

# THE AMERICAN
# MEDICAL ASSOCIATION

# WOMEN'S
# HEALTH

Medical Editor
CHARLES B. CLAYMAN, MD

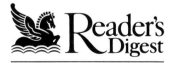

THE READER'S DIGEST ASSOCIATION, INC.
Pleasantville, New York/Montreal

The AMA Home Medical Library was created and produced
by Dorling Kindersley, Ltd., in association with the
American Medical Association.

The information in this book reflects current medical knowledge. The
recommendations and information are appropriate in most cases;
however, they are not a substitute for medical diagnosis. For specific
information concerning your personal medical condition, the AMA
suggests that you consult a physician.

The names of organizations, products, or alternative therapies appearing
in this book are given for informational purposes only. Their inclusion
does not imply AMA endorsement, nor does the omission of any
organization, product, or alternative therapy indicate AMA disapproval.

The AMA Home Medical Library is distinct from and unrelated to the
series of health books published by Random House, Inc., in conjunction
with the American Medical Association under the names "The AMA Home
Reference Library" and "The AMA Home Health Library."

**Library of Congress Cataloging in Publication Data**

Women's health / medical editor, Charles B. Clayman.
        p.  cm — (The American Medical Association home medical
library)
  At head of title: The American Medical Association.
  Includes index.
  ISBN 0-89577-398-8
  1. Women — Health and hygiene.  2. Women — Diseases.  I. Clayman,
Charles B.  II. American Medical Association.  III. Series.
RA778.W753 1992
613'.04244 — dc20                              91-15417

# FOREWORD

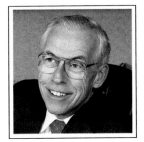

Women today have many more options open to them than their mothers and grandmothers did – and certainly those options include new ways of managing their health and medical care. Advances in medical testing, such as the Pap smear for cervical cancer and mammography for breast cancer, greatly reduce the risk of disease. Developments in the areas of contraception and fertility give women unprecedented control over their reproductive lives. Greater understanding of the importance of diet and exercise enables all of us to take better care of ourselves.

To benefit fully from today's medical knowledge, and to exercise their options wisely for themselves and their families, women have become well-informed and active participants in their health care. In this volume of the AMA Home Medical Library, we offer women of all ages up-to-date, reliable medical information. We have designed this book to give you a better understanding of your body and how it works and information to help you decide when to seek professional help for your symptoms and other problems. We have also suggested useful ways to work effectively with your doctor to get your questions answered and to prevent or manage illness.

To younger women – we hope this book helps you make informed decisions that will improve your health now and help determine how you look and feel in your later years. If you have reached mid-life or older, we hope to contribute to your vitality and confidence about your health by discussing ways in which you can manage the menopause and other life changes. Women of all ages need calcium and exercise to prevent osteoporosis. We offer ideas about how you can incorporate good nutrition and fitness into the way you live.

In the chapters of this book, we at the American Medical Association offer you the facts and guidance to help you enjoy the highest possible level of good health.

*James S. Todd MD*

**JAMES S. TODD, MD**
Executive Vice President
American Medical Association

# CONTENTS

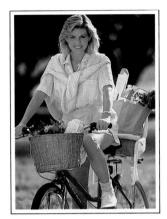

# CHAPTER ONE

# THE FEMALE LIFE CYCLE

NOT UNTIL the 20th century have large numbers of women truly been able to rewrite the roles that society has traditionally offered them. In many cultures throughout history, men have been considered the dominant sex. However, science has demonstrated that in many respects women have physiological advantages over men. Although, in general, men have greater physical size and strength, women have more stamina, are better at managing stress, have a greater resistance to disease, and have longer life spans. Today's women need all of these advantages – they often juggle professional, financial, social, and family responsibilities. In the past 40 years, the number of women entering the workplace has increased significantly. But most women go home from work to face the lion's share of the domestic and childcare duties.

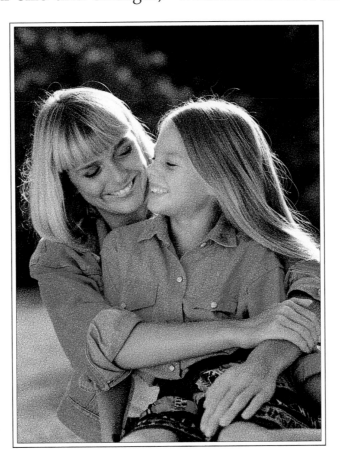

Until the advent of reliable forms of contraception, sexual intercourse before menopause posed the inescapable possibility of pregnancy. Before the introduction of antibacterial drugs and blood transfusions, every pregnancy carried the risk of death. As late as the year 1920, 5,000 women died during childbirth in the US. Of course, the risks associated with childbearing were an important influence on a woman's life ex-

pectancy. Historians estimate that the average life span for a woman in ancient Rome was 35 years, while the average life span for a man was 40 years. These figures remained stable until well into the 19th century. But times have changed. Advances in medicine and the introduction of successful screening programs for diseases such as breast cancer and cervical cancer have enabled women to monitor their health more closely, and the average woman's life expectancy is longer than ever before. Women in the 1990s live twice as long as their female ancestors did – to an average of 77 years. Women now outlive men by 5 years on the average.

Because their immune systems are more sensitive, women are more susceptible than men to autoimmune diseases such as rheumatoid arthritis. On the other hand, women experience fewer heart attacks and strokes than men. Until recently, women were at a much lower risk of alcohol-related and smoking-related illnesses than men were, largely because smoking and drinking were more common among men. In recent years, larger numbers of young women have been smoking and drinking. If that unfortunate trend continues, related health disorders will develop in women in ever-increasing numbers.

# A WOMAN IS BORN

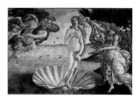

While many of the differences between women and men are obvious, their origins are still the subject of study. Some sexual differences are genetic, some are hormonal, and some are the result of social expectations. Until recently, sex roles in society were largely defined by physical size and strength. Many cultures rewarded women who were effective caregivers just as they rewarded men who were successful aggressors. Today, gender stereotypes are becoming more flexible. Recent research has focused on how girls and boys differ genetically and hormonally and why they behave differently, in some respects, from birth onward.

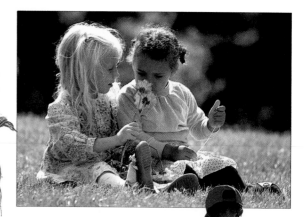

**From Botticelli to baseball**
*The demure goddess of love in Botticelli's Birth of Venus (left) represents a romanticized, passive vision of femininity that many now consider restrictive. Young girls today are likely to play baseball as wholeheartedly as they play with dolls (right).*

## SEX DETERMINATION

The sex of a child is determined at the moment of conception when an ovum (egg) is fertilized by a sperm. Whether the resulting embryo is female or male is a matter of chance, governed by the chromosomes – threadlike structures in the cell nucleus that carry genetic determinants – of the father's sperm. All ova carry X chromosomes; only some sperm carry a Y chromosome. An egg fertilized by an X sperm will develop into an embryo with two X chromosomes (XX) and will become female. If the egg is fertilized by a Y sperm, the embryo will have one X and one Y chromosome (XY) and will be male. Every embryo contains 23 pairs of chromosomes; 22 are the same in both sexes. The 23rd pair – the XX or XY pair – are called the sex chromosomes.

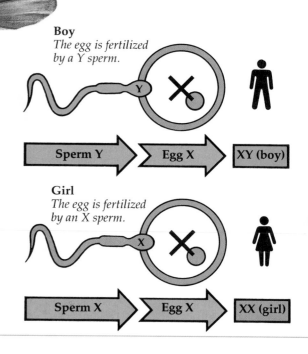

**Boy**
*The egg is fertilized by a Y sperm.*

| Sperm Y | Egg X | XY (boy) |

**Girl**
*The egg is fertilized by an X sperm.*

| Sperm X | Egg X | XX (girl) |

## STARTING AT CONCEPTION

Under a microscope, an X chromosome and a Y chromosome look completely different. The Y chromosome is believed to provide all the information for the development of male sexual characteristics. In its absence, the female pattern of development occurs.

### Sex ratios at birth

Ratios of female births to male births vary from country to country. In the US, this ratio is 100 females to 105 males, in Korea it is 100 to 115, and in Jamaica it is 100 to 103. Statistics show slight seasonal variations in birth ratios. Firstborns are more likely to be male, as are babies born to young mothers. Little is known about why these variations occur. X sperm are believed to survive longer than Y sperm and prefer an acid to an alkaline environment. Some doctors claim that the chances of a girl being conceived are higher when intercourse takes place 2 to 3 days before ovulation, when vaginal secretions are more acidic. Colorful folklore suggests that either a boy or a girl can be conceived by altering the diet, douching, or even positioning the body in a certain way during intercourse. None of these claims has ever been proven.

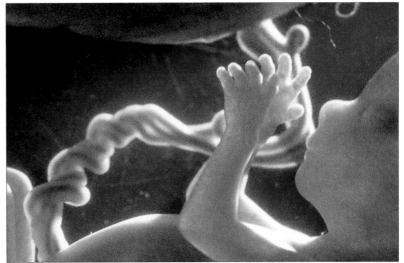

More males than females are conceived and born, but today higher male death rates from the first year of life onward offset this numerical headstart.

### Hormonal development

Recent research has revealed a specific gene on the Y chromosome that seems to determine biological maleness. This gene determines whether the early embryo develops testes or ovaries. All the remaining differences in development appear to depend on the hormones secreted by these sex glands during embryonic growth. The ovaries secrete the female hormones estrogen and progesterone. These are the hormones that, among other things, make women characteristically shorter and lighter than men, with smaller bones and muscles. The testes produce the male hormone testosterone. The effects of hormones on sexual development are illustrated by the rare testicular feminization syndrome. The embryo is a genetic male (one X and one Y chromosome) that develops testes and produces male hormone normally. However, none of the target organs responds to the male hormone, and normal male development is suppressed.

**Pairs of chromosomes**
*A healthy human cell contains 23 pairs of chromosomes, including the sex chromosomes. A male set (left) has one X and one Y sex chromosome. A female has two X chromosomes.*

**Is it a boy or a girl?**
*Techniques of chromosomal analysis, such as chorionic villus sampling and amniocentesis, are used to detect fetal abnormalities. These techniques also can reveal the sex of your embryo. Chorionic villus sampling, usually performed vaginally during the first 3 months of pregnancy, removes a sample of the placenta for chromosomal analysis. Amniocentesis is usually done in the fourth month. A needle is inserted through the abdomen into the uterus and a sample of amniotic fluid is withdrawn and analyzed. These readily available methods are now used to detect a fetus with a serious abnormality such as Down's syndrome. In such cases, termination of pregnancy may be considered.*

# A CHILD'S DEVELOPING BODY

From babyhood on, the differences between a girl and a boy become more pronounced. The stage of development during which a child makes the physical transition into adulthood is called puberty. Puberty usually begins at about age 11 in girls and about 2 years later in boys. The entire process takes about 3 to 4 years to complete for either sex. In addition to sex-specific changes, height and weight both increase rapidly. Puberty is complete when the girl or boy is capable of reproduction – that is, when ovulation or sperm production is occurring. The term adolescence refers to the entire period of development – emotional, intellectual, and physical – from childhood into adulthood. This complex transition continues for some time after puberty.

## EMOTIONAL CHANGES

The physical changes of puberty are accompanied by emotional changes that are also triggered by sex hormones. In both boys and girls, these hormones stimulate interest in sexuality and increase natural assertiveness. If a child's physical development is later than average, emotional maturity may also occur later. For a time, the child may have difficulties coming to terms with being smaller, less physically developed, and less assertive than his or her friends.

**The 11-year-old girl**
*At about age 11, a girl shows the first signs of puberty – usually an increase in height and weight. Her pubic hair appears and her breasts begin to form, starting with an increase in the size of the nipples.*

**The 11-year-old boy**
*At age 11, some boys may have some increase in the size of their testicles and possibly some pubic hair growth, but these changes are not as obvious as those taking place in their female counterparts.*

**The 7-year-old child**
*At age 7, girls and boys look somewhat similar except for their external genitalia. Their bodies are more or less the same shape, and the skin of both sexes has a covering of soft, downy hair.*

**The 14-year-old boy**
*The 14-year-old boy continues to develop – he is growing in height and weight at a dramatic rate, his shoulders and chest start to broaden, his trunk lengthens, and he usually has an increased appetite. As his larynx starts to enlarge, his voice deepens and an Adam's apple may be noticeable at the front of his neck when he swallows.*

**The 14-year-old girl**
*By the time a girl is 14, she has usually started her menstrual periods and has grown under-arm and pubic hair that gradually thickens and coarsens over the next few years. At the same time, the nipples darken and sweat glands become active under the arms, in the groin, and around the nipples.*

**The 17-year-old girl**
*By age 17, a girl's voice has gradually become mature, her hips have become wider and fuller (to accommodate pregnancy and childbirth), and her menstrual cycle is now regular. Her breasts are fully developed and puberty is over. She has reached sexual maturity.*

**The 17-year-old boy**
*At 17, a boy is showing most of the signs of adulthood. The skin of the scrotum darkens, the penis lengthens, and ejaculation of seminal fluid is usually possible. His pubic and underarm hair is now coarse and thick, and his facial hair is starting to grow. Depending on inherited characteristics, hair may also grow on other areas of his body, such as his chest, abdomen, and back. Sweat glands develop under the arms, in the groin, and around the nipples. Boys continue to grow and develop physically up to about age 20.*

## GROWTH RATES

Before puberty, girls and boys grow at approximately the same rate, and both sexes attain a median height of about 54 inches by age 10. The changes brought about by puberty lead to a dramatic increase in the rate of growth, although this occurs at an earlier age in girls than in boys. The growth spurt (in which the annual increase in height doubles) begins during the tenth year in girls and about 2 years later in boys. However, during this growth spurt, a girl may grow at a rate of 3 inches a year, whereas boys grow faster, reaching a rate of 4 inches a year. The combination of later male puberty, which gives boys an extra 2 years of childhood growth before the spurt, and the faster rate of growth during adolescence, causes most men to attain a greater adult height than most women.

**Differences at birth**
*Some pediatricians claim that behavioral differences are apparent even at birth – for example, that girls are more sensitive to delicate touch while boys are more active.*

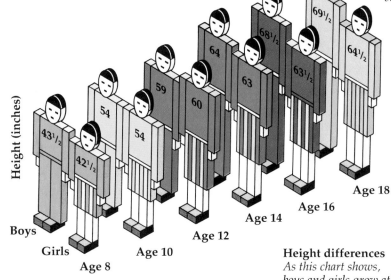

Height (inches)

43½  42½  54  54  59  60  64  63  68½  63½  69½  64½

Boys
Girls
Age 8
Age 10
Age 12
Age 14
Age 16
Age 18

**Height differences**
*As this chart shows, boys and girls grow at about the same rate up to the age of 10. A growth spurt gives girls a short-lived height advantage. By age 14, boys are usually taller than girls. From then on, boys gain steadily, on the average. Doctors often use growth charts to check whether growth is significantly above or below average.*

## DEATH RATES

Mortality in the first year of life is 25 percent lower for girls than it is for boys. It is not known why girls are less susceptible to and die less often of life-threatening illness at this age.

In early childhood, the susceptibility to illness in the two sexes balances out, although there are significant differences in the rates of accidents and psychiatric disorders. For example, girls are less likely to be killed or injured in accidents on the road, climbing trees, or in water. And autism, a serious psychiatric condition in which children fail to form relationships with others, is three times more common in boys than in girls.

## Psychological differences

In childhood, differences in more minor psychological and psychiatric disorders are also apparent. For instance, about 5 percent of children have a persistent problem with stuttering, but the disorder is about three times more common in boys than in girls. Reading difficulties such as dyslexia are also substantially less common in girls, as are hyperactivity and bed-wetting. Girls mature a year or two earlier than boys, which may explain their enhanced performance on intelligence tests. In the early teenage years, girls outperform boys academically for reasons that are unclear. At the same time, teenage girls have higher rates of anorexia nervosa (an eating disorder) and attempted suicide.

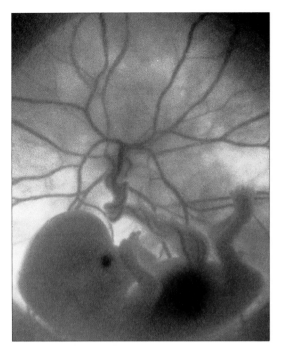

**Sexual development**
*By the 11th week of development (above), the sexual organs of a fetus have developed according to a genetically determined pattern of sex hormone secretion.*

amus initiates and maintains the cyclical pattern of female hormones that results in menstruation. In boys, it sustains the constant pattern of male sex hormone secretion. The complex differences between hypothalamic function in women and men are not yet fully understood.

## Sexual orientation

Some biologists have found evidence that hormonal influences on the brain during embryonic development may play a significant role in determining an individual's sexual orientation – that is, whether he or she is sexually and emotionally attracted to members of the opposite sex or, as is the case with about 10 percent of the world population, the same sex (homosexuality). These conclusions are still unconfirmed and controversial. Prenatal factors are probably among a number of variables that influence sexual orientation in individuals.

**SEX AND BEHAVIOR**

Scientific debate continues about the causes of behavioral differences between girls and boys. The differences may in part be caused by the influence of sex hormones and in part by social conditioning. Some scientists claim that, in cultures where social expectations for each of the sexes are more similar, behavior is the same in boys and girls. Others maintain that, even in such cultures, sex hormones influence the children's behavior substantially.

## SEX HORMONES AND THE BRAIN

Early in fetal development, the sex glands (ovaries or testes) start to secrete female or male sex hormones. These hormones control the development of female or male sex organs. The sex hormones also cause the hypothalamus, the part of the brain that governs hormone production, to secrete the hormones appropriate to the sex of the fetus. There are three main types of sex hormones – androgens (male sex hormones), estrogens (female sex hormones), and progesterones (hormones that have the specialized function of preparing a woman's body for and maintaining pregnancy). In girls, the hypothal-

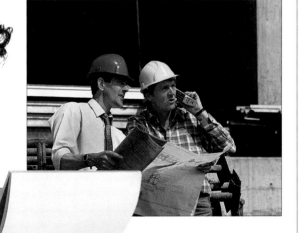

**Differing skills**
*It has been demonstrated that women on the average perform slightly better than men on intelligence tests requiring language skills (verbal ability), whereas men on the average perform slightly better than women on tests requiring visual/spatial skills such as solving problems involving pictures and three-dimensional models. The reasons for this are still being investigated.*

# THE FERTILE YEARS

Every woman can probably remember the start of her first menstrual period – how old she was, where she was, who she was with, and how she felt. Her memories are well placed because, among all the signs of growing up, a girl's first menstrual period is a clear signal in her biological life. Her young adult body is capable of reproduction.

## THE MENARCHE

The onset of menstruation is called the menarche, which is Greek for "month" and "beginning." A girl's first menstrual period is her first experience of the monthly shedding of the endometrium (the glandular lining of the uterus), which takes place if she does not become pregnant. The onset of menstruation signals the beginning of ovulation, the release once a month of a mature egg (ovum) from the ovary, which occurs midway through the menstrual cycle. A young woman's menstrual periods may not settle down to a regular monthly cycle for as long as 2 years after the menarche.

The age of the menarche varies among individuals and from one culture to another. It occurs in some girls as early as age 10 and in others as late as age 17. In the US, the typical age is about 12 or 13. The duration of the menstrual cycle once it is established also varies widely among women. The monthly cycle may take as little as 20 days in one woman and as long as 42 days in another.

## Sex education

A full explanation of menstruation is an excellent way to help a young girl develop a healthy, positive attitude toward her body and her sexuality. Because the age at which girls first experience the changes of puberty is so variable, and the initial menstrual cycles are likely to

**Breasts**
*The breasts are fully developed and the nipples are larger and darker in color than they were throughout adolescence. The breasts consist mainly of fat and are divided internally into about 20 lobes. Each of these lobes is traversed by a duct, which opens into the nipple. The ducts are connected to spaces called alveoli, which multiply and enlarge to produce milk when a woman becomes pregnant. The breasts are supported by ligaments. The female breast comes in all shapes and sizes and it is common for a woman to have one breast that is larger than the other.*

**Reproductive system**
*The female reproductive organs consist of a pair of ovaries linked to the uterus by two fallopian tubes. The base of the uterus forms the cervix, the lower part of which is enclosed by the upper part of the vagina. The vagina is about 4 inches long and opens to the outside of the body.*

**Muscles**
*A woman's muscles tend to be smaller and less powerful than those of a man.*

**Voice**
*A woman's larynx is smaller than that of a man, which is why her voice is higher pitched.*

**Body hair**
*Women generally have less hair than men, but most women have some hair around their nipples, under their arms, on their legs, and in their pubic area. Distribution of body hair varies widely among racial groups.*

**Bones**
*A woman's bones are lighter, smaller, and less dense than a man's.*

**Arms**
*A woman's arms are shorter and her forearms are more cylindrical. The angle at her elbow between her upper arm and forearm is more pronounced.*

**Hips**
*A woman's hips are as broad or broader than her shoulders and her waist is often comparatively narrow. By contrast, the waist and hips of a man differ little in width.*

**Legs**
*Compared to a man's legs, a woman's legs are shorter in relation to her trunk. The circumference of the top of her thigh is larger than that of a man. The angle at her knee between her thigh and the lower part of her leg is more pronounced because of her wider hips.*

**Body fat**
*Women have a greater proportion of fat to muscle in body weight than men. Because of the effects of the hormone estrogen, this additional fat is distributed more or less evenly around the buttocks, thighs, abdomen, upper arms, and chest. A woman's face also has more fat, which gives it a more rounded appearance.*

be erratic, it is important to give a young girl adequate information at an early age. The importance of sex education is underscored by the large numbers of unplanned pregnancies that occur in girls who are in their early teens. The average age of the menarche has been falling steadily in developed countries, and it is now entirely possible for a girl as young as 10 to enter her reproductive years. Early sex education is an important means of helping her understand and choose among the many options she has before her during the adult years.

## SEXUAL MATURITY

Just as a girl's body changes as she approaches the onset of menstruation, so her body will change again as she nears the menopause. Many of the characteristics of her body during her fertile years are influenced by the monthly cycle of production of female sex hormones, estrogen and progesterone, which begins at puberty and stops at the menopause. When this hormone production stops, the parts of her body influenced by the cycle begin to shrink.

Individual women vary widely in features such as height, weight, breast size, body proportion, and fat distribution. It is important to remember that these variations in body type are normal. The basic shape of the mature woman has evolved so that she is well suited for her biological role of giving birth. Specifically, her pelvis must be large enough to permit passage of an emerging baby's head.

# FEMALE REPRODUCTIVE BEHAVIOR

Unlike other female primates, women have the ability to reproduce at any time of the year – they are not limited to specific mating seasons. The menstrual cycle allows a woman to become pregnant in any given month because an egg is released about once a month. Today, readily available and reliable contraception enables women to decide if they will have children and to plan the timing and number of children they choose to have. Women today also have greater freedom to combine their work lives with their family lives throughout their reproductive years.

POSTPONING MOTHERHOOD

The chart below shows both the drop in birth rate and the trend toward delayed motherhood that has occurred in the US compared to earlier decades. For example, in 1960, the early 20s were the peak age for child-bearing; in 1985, this peak moved to the late 20s.

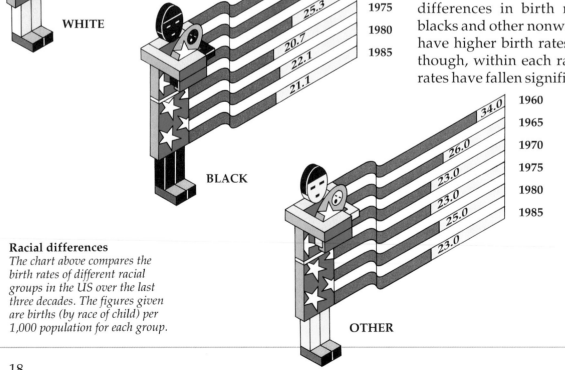

| | 1960 | 1965 | 1970 | 1975 | 1980 | 1985 |
|---|---|---|---|---|---|---|
| WHITE | 22.7 | 18.3 | 17.4 | 13.6 | 14.9 | 14.8 |
| BLACK | 31.9 | 27.7 | 25.3 | 20.7 | 22.1 | 21.1 |
| OTHER | 34.0 | 26.0 | 23.0 | 23.0 | 25.0 | 23.0 |

**Number of live babies per 1,000 women** — 250, 200, 150, 100, 50

Age   10-14   15-19   20-24   25-29   30-34   35-39   40-44   45-49

## A declining birth rate

In the US, the overall birth rate has fallen substantially and there has been a significant shift in the age at which women have their first child. There are also racial differences in birth rates. Generally, blacks and other nonwhite racial groups have higher birth rates than whites, although, within each racial group, birth rates have fallen significantly since 1960.

**Racial differences**
*The chart above compares the birth rates of different racial groups in the US over the last three decades. The figures given are births (by race of child) per 1,000 population for each group.*

## WOMEN AND DISEASE

Evidence shows that women are more resistant to stress-related diseases than men when exposed to the same stress-inducing situation. The difference is most apparent in studies of women and men who have particularly stressful occupations such as the medical, legal, and teaching professions. Women also appear to be better able to survive in extreme environmental conditions, although the precise reasons for their relative endurance are unknown. Women have stronger immune systems, which are probably stimulated by their female sex hormones. As a result, women are able to resist common infections, such as colds and influenza, more effectively than men. They also recover from any infections they do get more rapidly.

## Health disadvantages

A woman's relatively more efficient immune system has disadvantages as well as benefits. Many of the autoimmune diseases (those caused by the body's immune system reacting against its own tissues) are much more common in women. These autoimmune diseases include rheumatoid arthritis; pernicious anemia; systemic lupus erythematosus, one of a group of diseases that cause inflammation of the connective tissue in many systems of the body; and Graves' disease, a type of hyperthyroidism. These diseases are life-long and potentially debilitating, so a woman's more efficient immune system can be a double-edged sword.

## FEMALE ABILITIES

The adult woman's biological role as a childbearer has influenced (in many respects) how her body is constructed and how she performs certain tasks. The dif-

**Women in gymnastics**
*Women's gymnastics have developed into a more athletically aggressive sport in the last 20 years, probably reflecting changes in thought about women's physical capabilities. Many of the gymnasts who have captured attention worldwide – and have helped change the nature of the sport – are very young girls whose petite frames are ideally suited to the athletic demands of the exercises. Today, women gymnasts must develop great strength, flexibility, and speed to perform successfully.*

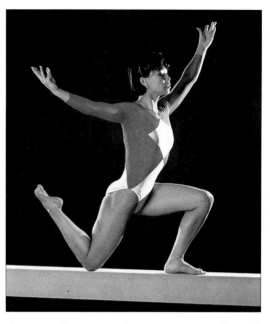

**Running times**
*Because the efficiency of a muscle partly depends on its mass, men tend to be faster runners than women.*

ferences between the two sexes in length of bones, muscle bulk, the carrying angle of the arms, width of hips, and body fat proportion dictate that women do not perform certain activities in the same way that men do. For example, the higher percentage of body fat in women means that they require little effort to stay afloat in water while men tend to sink more easily because of their denser bones and greater muscle bulk. However, in athletics, because of the physical differences between the sexes, the records for men's running and throwing events exceed the women's equivalents. As a result, athletic performances should be compared among women rather than between women and men. However, women are no longer excluded from competing in many events and women now compete equally with men in skill-oriented sports such as equestrian events where physical differences are less significant.

# THE MENSTRUAL CYCLE

Even at its most unpredictable, the female menstrual cycle is a striking example of hormonal clockwork. A number of processes take place simultaneously throughout the cycle, during which parts of the reproductive system and the hormonal system change and interact. Each month the entire process is poised to respond to the presence of a fertilized egg.

**Endometrium**

### INTERCOURSE DURING YOUR PERIOD

There is no medical reason to avoid sexual intercourse during your menstrual period. It is a "safe" time of the month if you wish to avoid pregnancy. The risk of contracting a sexually transmitted disease such as gonorrhea may be slightly greater during your period because the menstrual fluid is a good medium for bacterial growth. Use of a condom provides protection against bacteria. You can also wear a diaphragm when you have intercourse during your period; it will contain the menstrual fluid and provide a barrier against bacteria.

### Uterus
*The inner lining of the uterus is called the endometrium. The endometrium provides a thick layer of cells, rich in blood vessels, where a fertilized egg can implant. At the start of the menstrual cycle, estrogen stimulates the process of thickening the endometrium and both estrogen and progesterone continue to prepare the uterus for implantation. If the egg is not fertilized, the lining breaks down and is shed, together with the egg and some blood. Approximately 1 ounce of fluid is lost during this process.*

### Cervix
*In the first half of the menstrual cycle, the mucus produced by the cells of the cervix is clear and stringy. The mucus is formed by the unopposed action of estrogen. Once ovulation has occurred, progesterone is produced and the cervical mucus thickens and becomes opaque. This change is significant because sperm can pass through clear but not opaque mucus, and so sperm are prevented from entering the uterus shortly after ovulation has occurred.*

### Ovary
*Under the influence of follicle-stimulating hormone (FSH) circulating in the bloodstream, the maturing ovum (egg) develops inside a structure called a follicle. The follicle ruptures under the influence of a surge of luteinizing hormone (LH) from the pituitary gland and the egg is released enclosed in a layer of jellylike material. The remaining cells form into a mass known as the corpus luteum. This structure degenerates if fertilization does not occur and is maintained if a pregnancy results.*

**Cervix**

**Vagina**

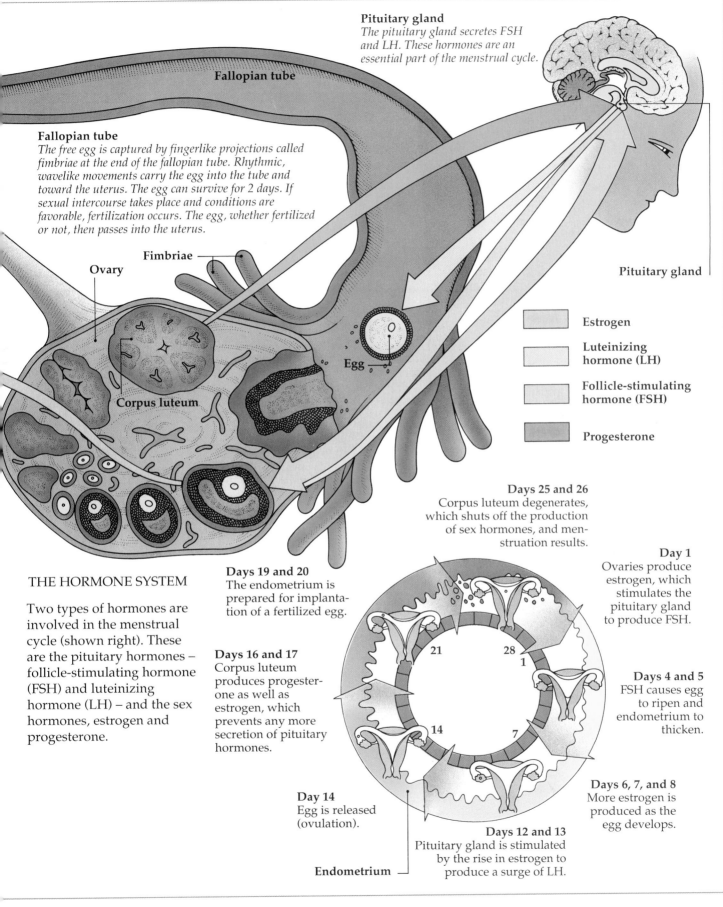

**Pituitary gland**
*The pituitary gland secretes FSH and LH. These hormones are an essential part of the menstrual cycle.*

**Fallopian tube**

**Fallopian tube**
*The free egg is captured by fingerlike projections called fimbriae at the end of the fallopian tube. Rhythmic, wavelike movements carry the egg into the tube and toward the uterus. The egg can survive for 2 days. If sexual intercourse takes place and conditions are favorable, fertilization occurs. The egg, whether fertilized or not, then passes into the uterus.*

**Fimbriae**

**Ovary**

**Pituitary gland**

**Egg**

Estrogen

Luteinizing hormone (LH)

Follicle-stimulating hormone (FSH)

**Corpus luteum**

Progesterone

**Days 25 and 26**
Corpus luteum degenerates, which shuts off the production of sex hormones, and menstruation results.

## THE HORMONE SYSTEM

Two types of hormones are involved in the menstrual cycle (shown right). These are the pituitary hormones – follicle-stimulating hormone (FSH) and luteinizing hormone (LH) – and the sex hormones, estrogen and progesterone.

**Days 19 and 20**
The endometrium is prepared for implantation of a fertilized egg.

**Days 16 and 17**
Corpus luteum produces progesterone as well as estrogen, which prevents any more secretion of pituitary hormones.

**Day 1**
Ovaries produce estrogen, which stimulates the pituitary gland to produce FSH.

**Days 4 and 5**
FSH causes egg to ripen and endometrium to thicken.

**Days 6, 7, and 8**
More estrogen is produced as the egg develops.

**Day 14**
Egg is released (ovulation).

**Days 12 and 13**
Pituitary gland is stimulated by the rise in estrogen to produce a surge of LH.

**Endometrium**

21

# PREGNANCY AND CHILDBIRTH

## HAVING A BABY

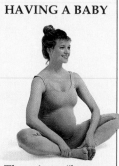

There is no "best age" at which to have a baby. Women in their late teens and early 20s may be at their physical peak but are often unable to cope financially or emotionally with the responsibility of a child. Many women consider the late 20s or early 30s (when fertility levels are still high) the best time for childbearing. After age 35, fertility starts to diminish, and the risk increases of having a miscarriage or a baby with an abnormality. These risks are greater after age 40, particularly the risk of having a baby with Down's syndrome. Techniques such as chorionic villus sampling and amniocentesis can detect fetal abnormalities early (see page 11). Yet most women over 40 have uncomplicated pregnancies and deliver healthy babies.

For most women, the joy of pregnancy is coupled with a strong sense of the responsibility they have assumed for the human life within them. To make sure that you are providing your baby with the best possible chance for healthy development, there are several steps you can take before and during your pregnancy. Many factors contribute to the health of a baby, but two of the most important and controllable factors are your nutrition and fitness. Prepregnancy planning is very important, and you should pay close attention to your diet and life-style before as well as after conceiving.

**Eating wisely**
*Before your pregnancy, make sure that you are eating a balanced diet, with plenty of fresh fruit, vegetables, fiber, fluids, and adequate amounts of protein. It is important that you continue to eat a healthy diet throughout your pregnancy.*

**Quitting smoking**
*Smoking is extremely harmful to you and your developing baby. You and the fetus can also be harmed by secondhand tobacco smoke.*

## PREPARING FOR CONCEPTION

It is ideal to begin thinking seriously about your health 3 to 6 months before you begin trying to conceive. If you are taking medications, check with your doctor to be certain that it is safe to continue their use during your pregnancy. Avoid all other drugs, including alcohol. Remember that plenty of sleep, a balanced diet, and exercise are important. You should ask your doctor to check that you have immunity against German measles. Couples with a family history of genetic diseases may be advised to obtain genetic counseling before conceiving.

**Planning together**
*Every couple thinking about starting a family should discuss fully the implications of parenthood. Both parents are undertaking a shared responsibility. A child can bring changes in household finances, a significant reduction in leisure time, and a dramatic change in life-style – both personal and professional.*

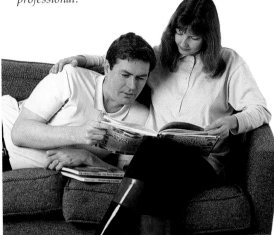

## MISCARRIAGE

About 10 to 20 percent of pregnancies end in miscarriage before the 28th week of pregnancy. The true figure may be even higher because any late, heavy period in a sexually active woman may be an undiagnosed early miscarriage. Most miscarriages occur in the first 3 months of pregnancy and are caused by abnormal development of either the fetus or the placenta. Study shows that more than half of these miscarried fetuses have a chromosomal abnormality originating in the sperm or the ovum, or during the process of fertilization.

Early miscarriage may also be caused by other conditions, such as a hormonal imbalance that causes the lining of the uterus to develop insufficiently or faulty development of the placenta. Both of these conditions result in the fetus being inadequately nourished. Other factors, including infections, can cause miscarriage. Any couple who experiences more than two miscarriages should seek medical help before conceiving again.

## LATE MISCARRIAGE

Miscarriage at any time and particularly late in pregnancy can have a profound effect on a woman and her partner. The woman experiences not only deep sadness associated with the loss of the baby but also emotional turmoil caused by the sudden drop in hormone levels. Some degree of depression is common, and professional help may be needed if the depression is prolonged. Miscarriage later in pregnancy has a variety of causes.

**Incompetent cervix**
*If the cervix has been damaged (for example, during a previous delivery), the muscles of the cervix may be unable to keep the cervix closed. This condition can result in a miscarriage, typically around the 20th week. However, your doctor may be able to prevent subsequent miscarriages by making a stitch around the cervix to keep it closed (right).*

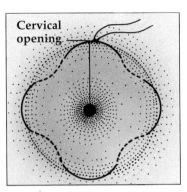

Cervical opening

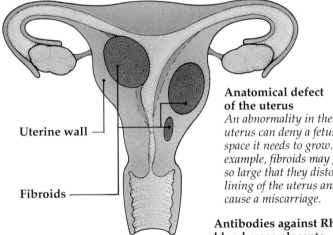

Uterine wall

Fibroids

**Anatomical defect of the uterus**
*An abnormality in the uterus can deny a fetus the space it needs to grow. For example, fibroids may grow so large that they distort the lining of the uterus and cause a miscarriage.*

**Antibodies against Rh+ blood cross placenta**

**Rhesus incompatibility**
*If a woman of the Rhesus negative (Rh-) blood group has a baby with Rhesus positive (Rh+) blood, her immune system becomes sensitized to Rh+ blood. During a subsequent pregnancy involving a fetus with Rh+ blood, the mother will form antibodies against the blood of the fetus, causing severe fetal anemia or death. This problem is now rare because mothers who have Rh- blood are immunized to prevent sensitization to Rh+ blood.*

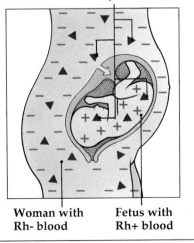

Woman with Rh- blood

Fetus with Rh+ blood

# THE CHANGES OF PREGNANCY

Throughout your pregnancy, you will notice a series of changes in your physical and mental state. Although some of these changes may be unpleasant, each one contributes to the intricate process of making your baby. Regular visits to your doctor are important during pregnancy. Strict dental hygiene and regular appointments with your dentist are also important while you are pregnant because your gums become more susceptible to infection. Monitor your weight carefully throughout your pregnancy; any extra pounds you gain while pregnant are just as difficult to lose once you have had your baby as weight gained at any other time.

## THE FIRST TRIMESTER (MONTHS 1 TO 3)

### Early hormonal changes
*Although some women experience no symptoms for weeks after conception and do not even realize that they are pregnant, others know that they are pregnant almost at once. These women are alerted by early onset of the symptoms described below and other changes in mental and physical well-being caused by the sudden increase in hormone levels. As the body adapts to the hormonal changes, these early symptoms fade, and most pregnant women begin to feel much better by the 12th week. However, for many women, it is encouraging to know that the first trimester is often the most difficult.*

### Nausea and vomiting
*One of the classic symptoms of early pregnancy is so-called morning sickness (vomiting). However, some women have this symptom at other times of the day and some experience no sickness at all.*

### Tiredness and dizziness
*Many women feel tired and lethargic during the early stages of pregnancy and some have occasional sensations of dizziness and faintness.*

### Changes in the breasts
*Very early in pregnancy, your breasts may start to feel full. Further into the first trimester, they often become sore and tender.*

### Increased urination
*You may find that you need to urinate more frequently in response to the dramatic changes in your hormone levels.*

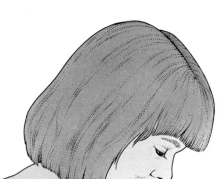

## THE SECOND TRIMESTER (MONTHS 4 TO 6)

### The pregnancy "bloom"
*During the middle months of pregnancy, most women feel quite well. The tiredness and nausea of the first trimester often disappear and are replaced by a surge of energy and a feeling of contentment.*

### Effect on the stomach
*In the middle trimester, the increased bulk of the uterus pushes the contents of the abdomen upward, causing indigestion. There may also be a reflux of gastric acid from the stomach into the esophagus, causing heartburn. You may be able to reduce these symptoms by modifying your diet and avoiding large, rich, or high-fat meals. Your doctor may suggest an antacid medication to reduce your heartburn.*

### Effect on the intestines
*Constipation may be a problem in the second trimester, and a high-fiber diet with liberal fluid intake is recommended as a preventive measure. Do not take stimulant laxatives because they can cause the uterus to contract. The pressure of the enlarging uterus on the pelvic organs can also cause hemorrhoids, and straining to pass a hard stool may worsen the condition. Your doctor can prescribe a stool-softening agent to help you cope with this problem.*

# THE THIRD TRIMESTER (MONTHS 7 TO 9)

**Sleeping problems**
*You will probably become increasingly tired because the bulk of your abdomen, symptoms such as heartburn (especially when you are lying down), and an increased urge to urinate make it difficult to get adequate sleep.*

**Aches in the joints**
*The added weight of your baby places extra strain on all weight-bearing joints, so your hips and knees may ache.*

**Backache**
*In the third trimester, nearly all women experience some degree of backache, and some have pain radiating down the back of one or both legs caused by pressure on the sciatic nerves. To ease back pain, avoid high-heeled shoes and try to maintain an erect posture. When you are lifting heavy objects, bend your knees rather than your back so that your knees take the strain.*

**Heartburn**
*The heartburn experienced in the second trimester may become more severe, with increased pressure of the baby on the stomach.*

**Shortness of breath**
*Toward the end of the pregnancy, the pressure of the baby high in the abdomen can cause rib pain, and you may also experience shortness of breath because your diaphragm is restricted.*

**Increased urination**
*You have the urge to urinate more often because there is no longer room in your pelvis for a large volume of urine to be stored in the bladder.*

**Varicose veins**
*Varicose veins may start to appear on your legs as pressure on the large veins of the pelvis causes blood to pool in the veins of your legs. The varicose veins become more pronounced if you stand for long periods. Wearing support hose can help. Usually the condition improves after delivery.*

## OVERALL CHANGES

Changes in your hormone levels have beneficial effects on your skin, hair, and nails throughout pregnancy. However, the skin of your abdomen must stretch considerably and stretch marks may develop in spite of the improvements in skin quality brought on by your hormonal changes. Whether stretch marks develop or not depends largely on your skin type, and the marks are more likely to occur if you are young and overweight. Your hormone changes may also cause a distinct dark line to appear between your navel and your pubic hair. Increases in your hormone levels affect your emotional state too. You may find that you feel more moody, cry more, or feel unusually insecure. The change in your body shape may seem hard to accept but it is only temporary.

# PROBLEMS IN PREGNANCY

Although most women have uncomplicated pregnancies and deliver healthy babies, problems can occur. Such problems include bleeding during pregnancy, preeclampsia (a syndrome characterized by protein in the urine, swollen ankles, and raised blood pressure), diabetes, and premature labor.

## Bleeding in early pregnancy

If bleeding and cramping develop early in your pregnancy, seek medical advice immediately. Although these symptoms may be a warning of an early miscarriage, some women bleed early in pregnancy for no apparent reason and with no adverse effect on the developing fetus. Your doctor may recommend that you have an ultrasound scan. If there is no cause for concern, you may be prescribed a period of bed rest. If the scan confirms that you are having a miscarriage, a dilation and curettage (D and C), a procedure in which the lining of the uterus is scraped away, may be required.

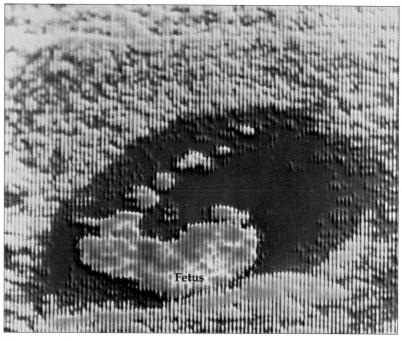

Fetus

**Ultrasound scanning**
*If you bleed in the first trimester, your doctor may recommend ultrasound scanning to determine that the pregnancy is not ectopic (occurring in a fallopian tube) and to ensure that fetal development is progressing normally.*

**Placenta previa**
*Placenta previa is a condition in which the placenta attaches to the lower segment of the uterine wall instead of the upper part. As the lower segment expands, there is painless bleeding from the placental attachment that, if heavy, can be dangerous for both mother and fetus. Women in whom placenta previa is diagnosed are usually prescribed strict bed rest and sometimes hospitalized for as much as the final 2 months of the pregnancy. If the placenta covers the opening of the cervix or partially obstructs the cervical canal, a cesarean section is performed.*

Misplaced placenta ———

Blocked cervix ———

Uterine wall

## Bleeding in late pregnancy

In the last 3 months of pregnancy, the two main causes of bleeding are related to the placenta. The first cause, called placental abruption, occurs when part of the placenta becomes separated from the wall of the uterus. Abruption is usually very painful and the uterus becomes hard. If a large area of placenta becomes separated, it can be fatal to both mother and baby; an emergency cesarean section is usually performed. The second cause of bleeding in late pregnancy is called placenta previa (see left).

## Hypertension

In some women, pregnancy can cause a rise in blood pressure. Women who had high blood pressure (hypertension) before pregnancy are most at risk of further elevation. High blood pressure is harmful to the fetus because it reduces the blood circulating through the placenta, which can retard fetal growth. Hypertension can almost always be controlled with one or more antihypertensive drugs. If hypertension occurs with fluid retention (edema) and protein in the urine, a condition called preeclampsia results. Preeclampsia is most likely to occur during a first pregnancy. If your doctor diagnoses preeclampsia, he or she may prescribe bed rest, hospitalization, and/or deliver your baby early. If preeclampsia is not treated, it can lead to the more severe condition of eclampsia. Blood pressure can become dangerously high, severely endangering the fetus or causing placental abruption (see page 26), or a stroke or seizures in the mother.

## Diabetes

Although most women with diabetes have normal pregnancies, problems can occur if their diabetes is not carefully controlled. Diabetes can also develop for the first time as a result of the metabolic and chemical changes of pregnancy; your doctor may test your urine for sugar during each prenatal visit for this reason. Poor control of diabetes at and around the time of conception increases the risk of fetal malformation. Later in pregnancy it may cause the baby to grow faster and larger than normal. This can lead to difficulties at birth. Sometimes the blood sugar level can be controlled by diet alone. However, daily injections of insulin are sometimes required.

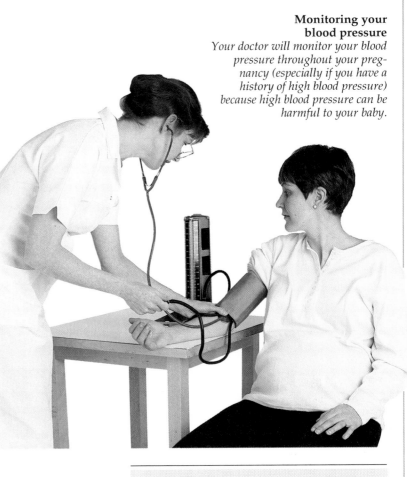

**Monitoring your blood pressure**
*Your doctor will monitor your blood pressure throughout your pregnancy (especially if you have a history of high blood pressure) because high blood pressure can be harmful to your baby.*

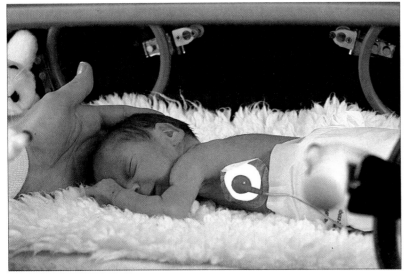

**Premature labor**
*Premature labor is defined as labor that begins before 37 weeks of gestation. In about 40 percent of cases, the cause of the early onset of labor is not known. Rest and medication will often help to quiet uterine activity. With the correct care and facilities, babies born after only 25 weeks of gestation can now survive.*

## RECOGNIZING LABOR

Most pregnancies proceed without complication to about 40 weeks, when true labor begins. Warning signs include a thick, bloodstained discharge; a release of the amniotic fluid around the fetus (known as the waters); and strong, frequent, long uterine contractions.

During the first stage of labor, the cervix slowly dilates to allow the passage of the baby's head into the vagina. This stage is the longest and can last up to 12 hours. During the second stage of labor, the cervix is fully dilated and the baby moves down the vagina, aided by the mother's pushing, until it emerges. The third and final stage involves the passing of the placenta after the baby is born. An injection is often given to speed up this process by helping the uterus contract. This injection also helps to prevent heavy bleeding after the delivery.

# TYPES OF DELIVERY

A pregnant woman can discuss with her doctor several possible methods of delivery. The method chosen usually depends on a combination of factors. A woman may consider her own physical condition, the condition of her baby, and her feelings about delivering the baby without the use of anesthetics. In the US, 98 percent of deliveries now occur in a hospital setting. Many hospitals have eliminated formerly routine procedures such as episiotomies, enemas, and shaving the hair around the anus when these procedures are not required for medical reasons.

## PAIN RELIEF DURING LABOR

Pain relief may be necessary during labor if your pain interferes with your ability to push hard and effectively in the later stages of labor. Several forms of pain relief are currently available. Several childbirth training programs teach women to cope with labor pains through emotional preparation for the labor experience and relaxation techniques in order to avoid any unnecessary use of pain medication.

### Analgesics
*Drugs used to relieve the pain of women in labor include nitrous oxide, which is an inhaled gas, and some injected narcotics related to morphine. Narcotics can cross the placenta and cause breathing difficulties for the baby at birth, so their use has diminished. Today, narcotics are used only with care in the later stages of labor.*

### Anesthetics
*Epidural anesthesia is a common technique for pain relief during labor and delivery. A thin catheter is inserted into the lower part of your back and a local anesthetic is injected, causing numbness from the waist down (sometimes into your thighs) and providing complete pain relief. The anesthetic is often allowed to wear off after earlier, more painful stages of labor so that you have energy for pushing.*

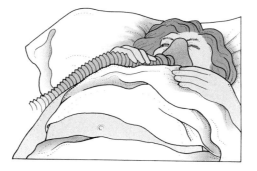

**Area affected by the epidural**

**Base of spine**

### Other techniques
*Other forms of pain relief include local pudendal (genital) blocks, which are injections of anesthetic that block the nerves of the groin area (usually used for forceps deliveries), and local anesthetic for the wall of the vagina (used before episiotomy).*

**Pudendal nerve**

### Uncomplicated vaginal delivery
*Most women give birth through the vagina. Involuntary uterine contractions push the baby out of the uterus, usually head first. Then the mother's deliberate pushing actions move the baby out of the vaginal opening.*

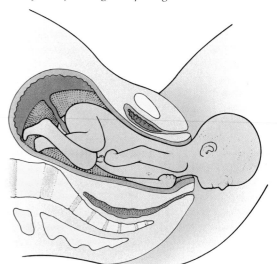

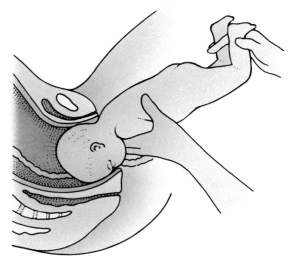

### Breech birth
*A breech birth is one in which the baby is born buttocks first. Most babies are in the breech position in the uterus until about the 32nd week of pregnancy, when they turn upside down on their own. However, 2 to 3 percent of babies remain in the breech position at the time of birth. There is an increased risk of birth injuries to babies born vaginally in the breech position, although this risk is minimal if the baby is of average size and labor goes smoothly. Some physicians recommend cesarean section deliveries for all babies who are in the breech position. Other physicians recommend turning the baby – a procedure called external version. Still other obstetricians believe that a vaginal breech delivery is acceptable.*

## Forceps delivery

*Forceps are curved, metal instruments designed to fit around a baby's head to aid delivery. Your doctor uses forceps if you cannot push the baby out yourself, if the baby's head is sideways, if the baby is in distress or is very premature, or sometimes if the baby is in a breech position. The doctor firmly pulls the baby's head down the vagina with the forceps; once the head is delivered, the forceps are removed and the delivery is assisted by hand. Forceps can damage the birth canal and are used only when necessary.*

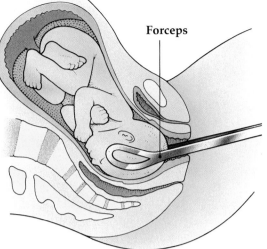

Forceps

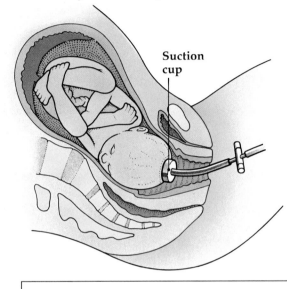

Suction cup

## Vacuum extraction

*Some obstetricians use vacuum extraction as an alternative to forceps delivery. The procedure is performed using an instrument called a vacuum extractor, which consists of a suction cup attached to a vacuum pump. Your doctor places the cup on the baby's head in the birth canal, turns on the vacuum pump, and then uses the instrument to pull the baby gently with each contraction. This delivery is usually slower than one using forceps, but it is gentler than a forceps delivery and does not necessarily require an episiotomy.*

## EPISIOTOMY

An episiotomy is a surgical incision into the woman's vagina to enlarge the opening and facilitate delivery. If the baby's head appears and it becomes apparent that birth will tear the vaginal tissue, the doctor makes a cut using scissors and a local anesthetic. The cut may be easier to repair and quicker to heal than a large vaginal tear. Episiotomies are performed to avoid pressure on the heads of babies who are in distress or are born prematurely, and are almost always done during forceps deliveries to prevent the forceps from tearing the vagina. Some women choose not to have an episiotomy performed if it is not necessary because the cut is painful immediately after the birth.

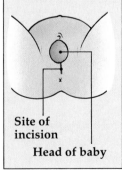

**Site of incision**

**Head of baby**

## CESAREAN SECTION

A cesarean section is a surgical operation in which the doctor delivers the baby from the uterus through an incision in the abdomen. The operation may be planned before labor starts if the baby is in the breech position, if the upper portion of the uterus is scarred from a previous cesarean, or if there is an infection of the vagina (such as genital herpes) that could affect the baby. Cesarean section is also used as an emergency procedure in situations such as fetal distress. In recent years, the number of cesarean sections performed in the US has risen. Approximately 25 percent of all babies in the US are now delivered by cesarean section as compared to 5 to 6 percent in European countries. Doctors generally agree that 25 percent is too high a cesarean section rate. While there are many reasons for the high rate in the

US, it is generally attributed to a legal climate in which some doctors anticipate being sued if they deliver a "less-than-perfect" baby. In addition, advances in hospital facilities may have encouraged the performance of more cesareans for delicate, premature infants. Better fetal monitoring techniques may have led to a high rate of detection of fetal problems in labor.

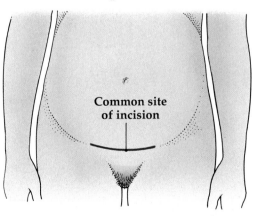

**Common site of incision**

# THE MENOPAUSAL YEARS

The last menstrual period of a woman's life marks the onset of the menopause. It signals the end of a woman's reproductive years, when she is no longer able to conceive and bear children. A woman's reproductive life begins when her ovaries start releasing eggs (ova) and the female sex hormone estrogen at puberty. The menopause occurs when estrogen production by the ovaries stops.

As a woman gets older, the supply of eggs in her ovaries diminishes and the ovaries gradually shrink. Estrogen production diminishes and the pituitary gland in the brain increases its output of follicle-stimulating hormone and luteinizing hormone (see THE MENSTRUAL CYCLE on page 20). These hormonal changes, particularly the reduction in the level of estrogen, are responsible for the physical changes that accompany the menopause.

## THE "CHANGE OF LIFE"

The cessation of periods is preceded by a transitional phase that may last a few months or even a few years. During this time, ovarian function begins to decline and ovulation becomes irregular; fertility is reduced. Symptoms related to the menopause can start during these years and also may occur during the 5 years or so after the menopause. The years surrounding the menopause are known medically as the climacteric. Many women refer to this time as the "change of life."

**Onset of the menopause**
*For most women, the menopause occurs between the ages of 48 and 52. Overall, the range is much wider; the menopause may occur as early as 39 or as late as 58. A woman goes through the menopause early if she has her ovaries removed or has received radiation therapy to the ovaries. Smokers and underweight women tend to have an earlier menopause while overweight women may have an early onset of menstruation and a later menopause. A woman tends to go through the menopause at about the same age that her mother did.*

## TREATING THE SYMPTOMS OF MENOPAUSE

Many women pass through the menopause without any significant problems. However, some need treatment, either to relieve
distressing symptoms or because some women (generally thin,
sedentary white women) are at high risk of osteoporosis. Other
women seek treatment because they wish
to prevent the long-term effects of
estrogen deficiency. Every woman
should be aware of the choices that are
available to meet her individual needs.

**Treatment options**
*The best-known treatment for menopau-
sal symptoms is hormone replacement
therapy (see page 34). Other treatments are available for specific
symptoms. Your doctor may
prescribe clonidine or an anti-
cholinergic (a drug that acts on
your autonomic nervous system)
for hot flashes, or you may
benefit from taking vitamin E
and from exercising. Lubri-
cants help treat vaginal
dryness. If you are at risk of
osteoporosis, the drugs
calcitonin and etidronate
may be prescribed for you.*

## Physical changes

In the years preceding the menopause,
changes occur in the regular monthly pattern of hormonal secretion and ovulation,
resulting in disruption of the menstrual
cycle. Deficiency of estrogen causes physical symptoms such as hot flashes, night
sweats, and vaginal dryness in about
75 percent of menopausal women. Estrogen deficiency also leads to physical
changes, including shrinkage of sex organs, some degree of osteoporosis (weakening of the bones), and an increased susceptibility to some types of heart disease.

## Psychological changes

In addition to the significant physical
changes that the menopause brings, some
women experience psychological and
emotional upheaval. Psychological problems that occur around the menopause are
not, however, always due to estrogen deficiency. You may be dealing with important
changes in your family, social life, or career

during these years. For example, if you
have children, they are likely to be young
adults who are leaving home. If your parents are still alive, they may be increasingly dependent on you as they grow older.

## Expectations and outlook

Although the menopause may cause some
temporary uncomfortable symptoms for
some women, other women find that their
postmenopausal years bring new personal
freedom and opportunities. Most women
do not miss the monthly inconvenience of
menstrual periods or the need to prevent
unwanted pregnancy. The end of the reproductive years may also signal the tapering
off of child-rearing responsibilities.

As you approach the menopause, think
carefully about the possibilities for your
life, and consider your life-style as it influences your health. Planning for your later
years is always useful, particularly if you
are considering moving to a different location or making job or family adjustments.

# HOW DO I RECOGNIZE THE MENOPAUSE?

Women vary considerably in the degree to which they are affected by menopausal symptoms. The questions below will give you an idea of the types of symptoms that you may – or may not – experience. The more "yes" answers you give to the questions, the more you may benefit from medical treatment. If you begin to notice symptoms, do not be concerned. The menopause is a natural stage in a woman's life. If your symptoms are troublesome, seek medical advice. As you read these questions, remember that, for many women, these symptoms are mild or absent.

## 1.

### Have you noticed any change in your periods?

In the 2 to 3 years leading up to the menopause, four of every five women notice changes in the frequency, duration, or regularity of their periods. These changes are usually the first sign that the menopause is approaching.

## 2.

### Do you have hot flashes?

Hot flashes are sensations of intense heat, sometimes with redness and sweating, that typically start in the chest and spread up the neck and face. Individual patterns may vary. About 70 percent of menopausal women experience hot flashes, sometimes for several years.

## 9.

### Have you lost interest in sex?

You may be reluctant to have intercourse if it is painful because of vaginal changes. Sex drive can decrease for other reasons, including hormonal changes, fatigue, and possible changes in your feelings about your partner.

## 10.

### Are you having difficulty sleeping?

You may have difficulty sleeping because of night sweats, hot flashes, and troubling emotions.

## 11.

### Have you experienced any other unexplained symptoms?

Women who are going through the menopause may experience a variety of other symptoms, including joint pains and muscle aches.

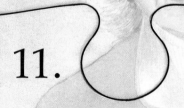

## 3.

**Do you sweat at night?**

Night sweats are a common menopausal symptom and may be so severe that you need to change your night-clothes or sheets.

## 4.

**Do you have vaginal dryness or irritation?**

Reduced levels of estrogen can cause the walls of your vagina to become thinner. The vagina itself can become shorter, narrower, drier, itchy, and more prone to infection.

## 5.

**Do you have dizziness and palpitations?**

Dizziness, headaches, and palpitations may occur as a result of changes in your circulation and heart rate.

## 6.

**Are you experiencing any urinary problems?**

Estrogen deficiency may affect your bladder and urethra, causing pain when you urinate, increased frequency of urination, and urinary incontinence.

## 8.

**Have you been feeling more anxious and irritable?**

Psychological symptoms such as anxiety, irritability, lack of concentration, and loss of confidence may be due to a combination of factors such as fluctuations in hormone levels, fatigue, and stress.

## 7.

**Do you feel depressed for no apparent reason?**

Some menopausal women experience depression or sudden changes of mood. These feelings may, in part, be caused by an estrogen deficiency, but you may also be responding emotionally to changing circumstances.

# HORMONE REPLACEMENT THERAPY

After the menopause, a woman's estrogen level is about 20 percent of her premenopausal level. Hormone replacement therapy gives you replacement estrogen, with or without a synthetic progesterone, to treat or prevent the problems that result from estrogen deficiency.

**Medical checkups**
*If you take hormones for more than a few months, make sure you have regular medical checkups, including breast and pelvic examinations and blood pressure measurements.*

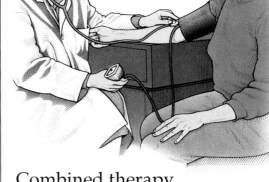

## REPLACEMENT HORMONES

Replacement hormones for menopausal symptoms come in a variety of forms, including tablets, injections, implants, skin patches, creams, and suppositories.

**Tablets**
*Hormonal tablets are taken by mouth, either every day or for 21 to 25 days each month.*

**Implants**
*Slow-release pellets of hormone are implanted, often under the skin of the abdomen. They are usually effective for 6 months to a year. These implants have not yet been approved for use in the US.*

**Skin patches**
*Skin patches containing a reservoir of hormone are applied to the skin, usually on the abdomen. The adhesive patch is replaced every 3 to 4 days at a slightly different site. The hormone is slowly absorbed from the patch through the skin into the bloodstream.*

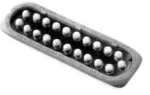

**Injections**
*Slow-release hormone injections into a muscle are given. Intervals between injections vary depending on the synthetic estrogen used.*

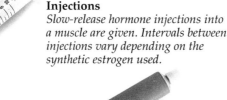

**Creams and suppositories**
*Topical preparations containing estrogen are used mainly to treat vaginal symptoms. The creams or suppositories are applied or inserted directly into the vagina one to three times a week to eliminate the symptoms of vaginal dryness.*

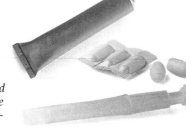

## Combined therapy

A number of the symptoms associated with the menopause are caused by your body's response to a decrease in your estrogen level. Hormone replacement therapy usually contains a form of progesterone as well as an estrogen, because estrogens taken alone can increase the risk of cancer of the endometrium (lining of the uterus). Usually, a synthetic progesterone is taken with the estrogen for 10 to 14 days each month. Bleeding occurs during the progesterone-free days of each month in the treatment cycle.

## Who should have hormone replacement therapy?

Some doctors recommend that women should take hormones only if menopausal symptoms – particularly hot flashes, night sweats, and vaginal soreness – are severe. Others believe that most women should take hormones to protect themselves against the effects of osteoporosis (weakening of the bones). Discuss the decision with your doctor.

## Monitoring the therapy

If you are taking hormones, you should have regular medical checkups, including pelvic examinations, cervical (Pap) smears, blood pressure checkups, and mammograms. Your doctor may evaluate any erratic bleeding or spotting, possibly with colposcopy, or with endometrial biopsy or endometrial aspiration.

## How long should treatment continue?

To eliminate symptoms such as hot flashes, most women require treatment for up to a year. If you stop treatment abruptly, the symptoms may return in a few months. To prevent osteoporosis, you may need to continue treatment for at least 5 to 10 years or indefinitely.

## Who should not have hormone replacement therapy?

Your doctor may advise you not to take hormones if you have had treatment for breast cancer or endometrial cancer. If you have liver disease, sickle cell anemia, or a history of embolism (arterial blockage by a variety of particles in the bloodstream) or deep vein thrombosis (blood clotting), ask your doctor about the use of hormones. Women who are severely obese, have hyperlipidemia (elevated blood fat levels), or otosclerosis (a hearing disorder) or who are heavy smokers may also be advised against having hormone therapy.

## The choice is yours

Hormone replacement therapy improves the quality of many women's lives. However, its long-term effects are still uncertain and little is known about the cumulative effects of hormone therapy on women who have previously used hormonal contraceptives. Before you make a decision about taking hormones, you must carefully consider the risks and benefits. Discuss the options with your doctor and with other women and remember that the final choice is yours.

## BENEFICIAL AND ADVERSE EFFECTS OF HORMONE REPLACEMENT THERAPY

| DISORDERS | EFFECTS OF THERAPY |
|---|---|
| Hot flashes, sweating, vaginal dryness | Very effective for treatment and prevention in the short term. |
| Depression | May reduce incidence of depression and improve sleep patterns and sense of well-being. |
| Osteoporosis | Slows down rate of bone thinning if taken for several years. Studies suggest that, if taken for 5 years, incidence of hip fractures is reduced. |
| Wrinkles | Long-term use can help maintain quality of skin and breast tissue. |
| Heart disease | Estrogen alone protects against atherosclerotic heart disease and reduces heart disease by 50 percent. Addition of progesterone neutralizes some of the benefits. |
| Monthly bleeding | The return of monthly bleeding may be seen as a drawback. Newer regimens try to eliminate monthly periods but many women experience irregular spotting. |
| Minor side effects | May cause headaches, nausea, breast tenderness, bloating, weight gain, jaundice, and depression. Your doctor may lower your dose to eliminate side effects. |
| Endometrial cancer | Estrogen alone increases risk of endometrial cancer. Risk removed by addition of progesterone. Endometrial aspiration, an office procedure, can screen for precancerous changes in the uterine lining. |
| Breast cancer | Some studies suggest that estrogen may increase risk of breast cancer. It is not known if adding progesterone gives protection. |
| High blood pressure | May increase blood pressure, although this is unusual at the dosage levels currently used. |
| Thrombosis | High doses of estrogen increase the risk of thrombotic disorders (such as blood clots, strokes, or thrombophlebitis) but the low doses used today have little effect on blood clotting. |

# WOMEN AFTER 65

With the menopausal years behind her, the changes that take place in a woman's body are as much the result of the physical process of aging as they are the effects of a lower estrogen level.

## INDIVIDUAL AGING RATES

All women age differently and at different rates. How your body ages depends largely on your genes, but your general health is also a major factor. The aging process may be accelerated by life-style factors such as smoking, alcohol consumption, poor diet, obesity, lack of exercise, and excess exposure to sunlight.

### Psychological changes
A woman must adapt psychologically as she grows older, adjusting to children leaving home, her retirement or the retirement of her partner, or, perhaps, to a new role as a grandmother. She may eventually have to care for an increasingly dependent partner or family member and she may someday become more dependent on others herself.

The ease with which a woman adapts to growing older depends not only on her health and circumstances but also on her own perception of age and aging. Research shows that both women and men remain functionally independent longer if they maintain a substantial degree of control over their living arrangements and have strong social ties with family and friends.

### Hormones and aging
After the menopause, the estrogen level in a woman's body is substantially reduced. The ovaries no longer produce estrogen but the adrenal glands, situated just above the kidneys, continue to make a small amount. Because of this fall in her estrogen level, a woman may find that

the hormone-related problems of her menstrual years – such as premenstrual tension, menstrual pains, and breast discomfort – finally disappear. The lack of estrogen does not diminish the need for regular gynecological examinations. A cervical (Pap) smear is recommended every 3 to 5 years. Older women are at increased risk of endometrial cancer; you need to seek treatment for any unexplained vaginal bleeding. Women over 65 should also have annual mammograms to check for breast cancer.

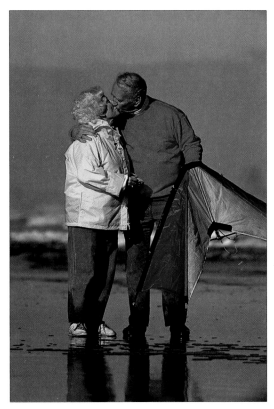

**Sex and the older woman**
*Many women continue to enjoy sexual activity through their later years. Some report finding sex more enjoyable in the years after the menopause, because they no longer have to worry about contraception and pregnancy. However, hormonal changes during and after the menopause can cause vaginal dryness; you may need to use a lubricant or take hormones to make intercourse easier. The availability of a sexual partner may be an important concern for the older woman, in part because women generally live longer than men.*

# THE PHYSICAL EFFECTS OF AGING

Your body undergoes a natural aging process during which there is a gradual deterioration of function and efficiency. Although you cannot avoid aging, there are steps you can take to slow down the rate or minimize the effects of this process.

**Brain and nervous system**
*A common reason for mental decline with aging is that people lose vital social or professional contact as they get older. You can stay mentally agile by keeping in touch with friends and colleagues and by increasing the amount of mental stimulation you receive through activities such as reading, traveling, or hobbies.*

**Cardiovascular system**
*The heart becomes less efficient and blood pressure rises with age. Arteries become less elastic and more prone to atherosclerosis (narrowing due to fatty deposits). Capillaries (tiny blood vessels) in the skin become more fragile, so that bruising occurs more easily. Smoking accelerates the development of disease in the cardiovascular system. However, if you are a smoker, it is not too late to quit – the risk of smoking-related diseases starts to diminish as soon as you quit.*

**Eyes and ears**
*The lenses in your eyes may become less elastic as you age; focusing on nearby objects may become more difficult. Some loss of hearing ability is also common because of degenerative changes in the inner ear. If your doctor recommends glasses or a hearing aid, don't be embarrassed to use them. They will help you function more effectively.*

**Genital tract**
*The vagina tends to become thinner and drier as you get older so it may be necessary to apply a lubricant to make sexual intercourse more comfortable. Pelvic floor muscles may lose their tone gradually.*

**Skeletal system**
*If osteoporosis develops as a woman grows older, her vertebrae can compress, leading to a loss of height and increased curvature of the spine. The bones lose density and become thinner and more liable to fracture. Weight-bearing exercise, including walking, bicycling, and stair-climbing, helps slow down the progression of osteoporosis.*

**Skin**
*Skin becomes thinner and more wrinkled as you get older due to loss of collagen, the protein that gives skin most of its elasticity. You should avoid excessive exposure to the sun throughout your life to reduce the destruction of elastic tissue. In addition to causing serious disease, smoking can speed up the development of wrinkles around the eyes and mouth and cause deep lines.*

**Muscles and joints**
*Muscles tend to lose their strength and bulk and tendons become less elastic as you get older. The protein collagen is modified in your joints and ligaments, resulting in stiffness and loss of mobility. Exercise can help reduce the effects of these changes, as well as help you avoid gaining weight. Exercise can also help prevent backache by keeping the muscles of the back and abdomen strong.*

## HEALTH PROBLEMS IN LATER LIFE

One of the consequences of aging is an increased susceptibility to disease. The three major causes of death in the elderly – heart disease, cancer, and stroke – become more common among both women and men. For women, some disorders – most notably osteoporosis (see WHAT IS OSTEOPOROSIS? on pages 130 and 131) and heart disease – occur at higher rates after menopause as a result of long-term reduction of estrogen.

### Coronary heart disease

Before age 50, the risk of coronary heart disease is about five times greater in men than in women. In other words, women before the menopause are much less likely to suffer from angina (chest pain caused by lack of oxygen to the heart muscle) or heart attacks than men of the same age.

## LIVING FOR HEALTH

Our individual susceptibility to disease is controlled partly by our genes, partly by our environment, and partly by our life-style. We cannot control our genes or many aspects of our environment, but we can make healthy choices about the way in which we lead our lives. A healthy life-style reduces the risk of premature death from heart disease and cancer and slows down the aging process.

**Healthy choices**
*You can influence the quality of your later years by following the principles of healthy living – eat sensibly, exercise regularly, don't smoke, limit alcohol consumption, minimize stress, maintain your weight at an appropriate level, and pay attention to safety both at home and on the road.*

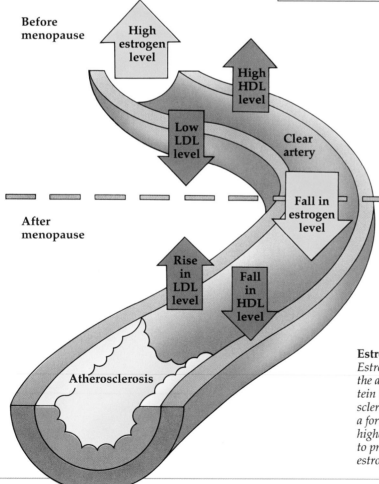

However, after the menopause, the incidence of coronary heart disease in women increases at a greater rate than it does in men. By age 65, women are as likely as men to have and to die of heart disease.

The risk of heart disease is increased in women who smoke, are overweight, have high blood pressure, or had close relatives die young of heart disease. The risk is also greater in women who went through the menopause early.

### Cancer

About half of all cancers occur in people older than 65; cancer is the second largest cause of death after heart disease in this age group. Before 65, the incidence of cancer in women and men is approximately equal;

**Estrogen and heart disease**
*Estrogen seems to help prevent atherosclerosis (narrowing of the arteries). Estrogen raises the level of high-density lipoprotein (HDL, a form of cholesterol that protects against atherosclerosis) and lowers the level of low-density lipoprotein (LDL, a form of cholesterol that contributes to atherosclerosis). The higher level of estrogen in women before the menopause seems to protect against coronary heart disease and the lower level of estrogen after the menopause seems to diminish this effect.*

from 65 onward, the incidence and death rates are higher in men than in women.

The increasing incidence of cancer with age is due to a variety of factors. The effects of a person's exposure to cancer-causing agents such as background radiation, cigarette smoke, sunlight, industrial or environmental pollutants (such as asbestos), and chemical toxins (such as industrial polyvinyls) are likely to accumulate and increase over time. Also, our immune systems gradually become less efficient at detecting and destroying any cells that have the capacity to develop into a benign or malignant tumor.

## Stroke

The incidence of stroke rises sharply with age. It is the third most common cause of death after heart disease and cancer. Almost 90 percent of women who have strokes are over 65. The main risk factor for stroke is high blood pressure. Other risk factors include a history of heart disease, diabetes mellitus, or high levels of cholesterol in the blood. Rehabilitation efforts enable many women to return to productive lives after a stroke. About half of all stroke patients recover more or less completely from their first stroke. A positive attitude is a significant factor in recovery.

**OBESITY**

Obese women have higher estrogen levels than trimmer women, so they are less prone to osteoporosis. However, they have higher rates of endometrial and breast cancer and are prone to high blood pressure, heart disease, stroke, diabetes mellitus, and osteoarthritis.

## CANCER DEATHS IN WOMEN AT VARIOUS AGES

The graph below shows how many women died, at different ages, of the most common types of cancers in the US in 1986. These figures do not reflect the incidence of cancer in women because many women survive cancers such as breast cancer and cervical cancer. Breast cancer is the most common type of cancer in older women, and its incidence increases with age. Cancers of the

female reproductive tract also increase with age. Endometrial and ovarian cancers are most common in women between the ages of 50 and 70. Cancer of the cervix reaches a peak rate at around age 50 and remains at a constantly high level from then onward. Cancers of the vulva and vagina, which can occur at any age after the menopause, are rare.

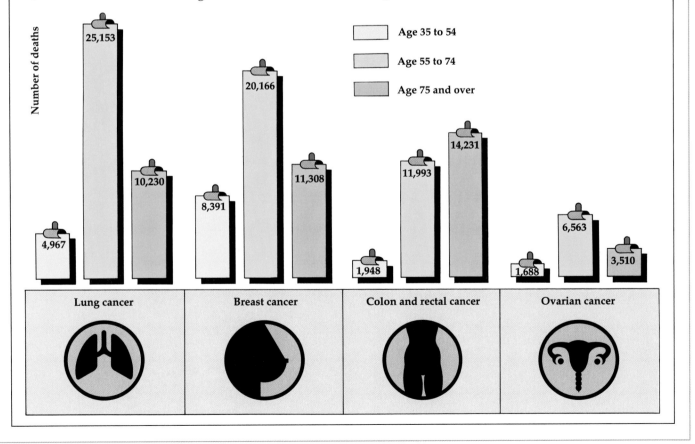

Number of deaths

□ Age 35 to 54
□ Age 55 to 74
□ Age 75 and over

Lung cancer: 4,967 / 25,153 / 10,230
Breast cancer: 8,391 / 20,166 / 11,308
Colon and rectal cancer: 1,948 / 11,993 / 14,231
Ovarian cancer: 1,688 / 6,563 / 3,510

# CHAPTER TWO

# STAYING HEALTHY

INTRODUCTION

DIET AND EXERCISE

MANAGING
YOUR OPTIONS

UNDERSTANDING
HEALTH HAZARDS

Y OUR BODY is an exquisite piece of machinery and your most valuable possession. You will enjoy life more if your body is fit and healthy. Over the past 20 years, millions of women have realized that preventive health care is the way to look and feel their best. These women are consciously making informed, positive choices to lead healthy lives and to protect themselves against factors now known to be harmful. This chapter provides information on what you can do to improve the state of your health and reduce your risk of certain diseases.

The first section emphasizes the importance of diet and exercise in maintaining good physical and psychological health. A nutritious diet has been shown to substantially reduce the risk of heart disease and stroke, and growing evidence demonstrates that it can also help protect you against

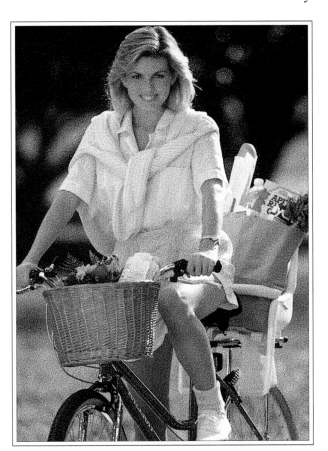

certain types of cancer. An extraordinary variety of appetizing meals can be prepared from ingredients that positively contribute to your health. You don't have to eat foods that you don't like just because they are healthy, and you need not completely deny yourself your not-so-healthy favorites. Nor is it necessary to force yourself to do tedious exercises every day. Choose an exercise that you enjoy and that you can incorporate into your daily life. You will soon begin to notice the many beneficial effects on both your body and your state of mind.

Stress is a fact of life. Everyone suffers from occasional stress but, in recent years, certain groups of women have become increasingly susceptible to stress-related disorders. Some researchers maintain that the hardest-working person in today's society, and the one most likely to experience damaging levels of stress, is a woman with a full-time job and one or more children. The section on managing your options explains what stress is and how to recognize the warning signs that you are under stress. It also offers some practical tips on how to deal with stress in different situations.

Finally, the section on understanding health hazards explains some of the precautions you can take to help you stay healthy well into your later years. While there are some potentially harmful factors that are outside your control even if you lead a healthy life, certain risks can be substantially reduced. Statistically, some of the most serious threats to the health of many Americans arise from avoidable factors such as smoking, heavy drinking, drug abuse, and irresponsible sexual activity. This section explains the consequences of each of these activities on your health.

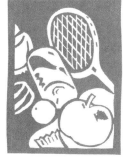

# DIET AND EXERCISE

**E**VERYONE BENEFITS from a healthy diet and regular exercise, and being in good shape can improve your quality of life and your self-esteem. But several aspects of diet and exercise are particularly relevant to women. For example, exercise and an adequate calcium intake can help prevent osteoporosis in later life.

It's not surprising that many women think about diet and exercise only as the means to a better figure. In fact, never-ending efforts to lose weight often contribute to nutritional deficiencies common in women (such as shortages of iron, calcium, folic acid, and zinc) and also to a lack of protein in their diets.

## BALANCING YOUR DIET

No single food is a threat to your health, as long as you don't eat too much of it. To help balance your diet, eat plenty of fresh fruits and vegetables, whole-grain breads and cereals, nuts, and dried beans. Try to choose foods that are low in fat, salt, and sugar and high in fiber. Choose low-fat red meats such as round or flank steak, and poultry such as chicken and turkey. Eat fish two or three times a week. Trim visible fat from meat and prepare by sautéing, roasting, or baking. Remove skin from poultry.

## WOMEN, FOOD, AND HEALTH

A healthy diet is one that provides a good balance of all the nutrients you need to stay healthy – carbohydrates, proteins, fats, vitamins, minerals, and fiber. In addition, to make sure that your weight stays in your optimum range, the amount of food energy (calories) that you consume should not be greater than the amount of energy you expend.

### Fats in your diet
Doctors are now certain that a high intake of fats, particularly saturated fats, can cause the accumulation of fatty deposits in our arteries (atherosclerosis). In time, these deposits cause a narrowing of the arteries, leading to an increased risk of coronary heart disease and stroke.

Saturated fat is the predominant type of fat in foods of

## FOOD SOURCES

**Fat**
*Skim or low-fat milk; low-fat yogurt and cheese; polyunsaturated and monounsaturated oils (found in olive oil and safflower oil)*

**Protein**
*Lean meat; poultry; fish; egg whites; skim or low-fat milk; low-fat cheese and yogurt; dried peas and beans; lentils; soy products such as tofu; nuts; cereals*

**Vitamins and minerals**
*Fresh fruits; fresh or frozen vegetables; fish; lean meat; poultry; skim or low-fat milk and other dairy products; whole-grain breads and cereals; soy products such as tofu; whole grains*

**Carbohydrates**
*Cereals; whole-grain bread, flour, and pasta; brown rice; potatoes; dried peas and beans; lentils; nuts; fruits; vegetables*

**Fiber**
*Whole-grain bread, flour, and pasta; cereals; brown rice; fruits; vegetables; dried peas and beans*

animal origin such as meats, butter, high-fat milk and cream, and in vegetable fats such as coconut oil and palm oil (found in processed snack foods) and cocoa butter (found in chocolate).

## Diet and disease

Obesity and too much salt in your diet can lead to high blood pressure. Reducing weight and salt intake benefits some people. Excessive alcohol consumption, particularly when combined with smoking; use of certain additives, such as nitrate and nitrite preservatives; use of smoked or salt-cured foods; a high-fat diet; and obesity have all been linked to different types of cancers. Some studies indicate that alcohol and excessive fat intake may contribute to breast cancer. A diet low in fiber may contribute to the development of intestinal disorders such as hemorrhoids and constipation and even to the development of cancer.

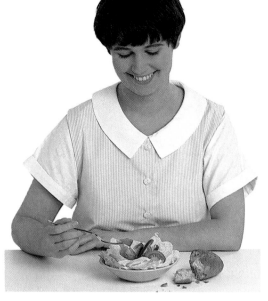

**Special needs for some women**
*Use of oral contraceptives may increase a woman's need for folic acid (found in green, leafy vegetables) and pyridoxine (found in chicken, fish, and bananas). During pregnancy, a woman's nutritional needs increase by about 10 percent. A woman who is breast-feeding needs some nutrients in still greater amounts to produce milk.*

### VITAMIN AND MINERAL SUPPLEMENTS

Women who are anemic from heavy periods may need to take an iron supplement. Many women should take calcium supplements if they do not drink milk or eat yogurt to reduce the risk of osteoporosis. Women on weight-loss diets and pregnant women may also need supplements. Ask your doctor about your need for supplements. Remember that you cannot rely on supplements to make up for poor eating habits.

## DIETING SENSIBLY

Studies show that most women believe they are fatter than they really are. However, if you are overweight, regular exercise and a balanced diet are the best ways to lose weight safely and permanently. To lose weight successfully without compromising your health, try following the advice below:

◆ Keep your calorie intake balanced throughout the day to avoid hunger, fatigue, and depression.
◆ Be aware of the nutritional composition of your foods. Choose foods that are rich in proteins, vitamins, and minerals to get the most nutrition for every calorie.
◆ Reduce the amount of fatty foods you eat. Unlike carbohydrate, dietary fat is stored directly in fat deposits around the body.
◆ Avoid alcoholic drinks; they are high in calories and have negligible nutritional value.
◆ Eat plenty of fiber to maintain bulk for good bowel function and drink large quantities of water to feel full.
◆ Smoking is not a good way to control weight. Smokers have more body fat as a percentage of body weight than nonsmokers.

**Are you overweight?**
*Use the chart (below) to calculate your body mass index. Place a ruler between your weight on the left and your height on the right, then read your body mass index from the middle scale. You are overweight if your body mass index is between 25 and 30 and obese if your index is over 30.*

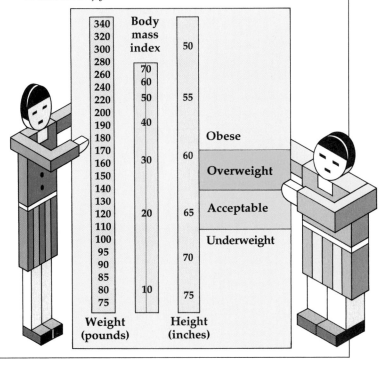

# WOMEN AND EXERCISE

The fitness boom of the past two decades has encouraged many women who had never before exercised regularly to enjoy the benefits of physical activity.

## Physical benefits

Exercising prepares your body for whatever demands you make of it; being fit helps your body perform more efficiently. Physically, exercise can improve your posture, reduce your risk of cardiovascular disease, improve the efficiency of your breathing, strengthen your muscles and bones, and help relieve premenstrual tension and menstrual pain. Regular exercise is even believed to help prevent some forms of cancer. If you are trying to lose weight, exercise is essential. It prevents loss of muscle protein, tones your muscles, curbs your appetite, and significantly increases your expenditure of calories.

## Mental benefits

You may discover that exercising improves your self-image and makes you feel more relaxed. During and immediately after exercise, you may experience a "high" caused by the release of natural morphinelike substances (endorphins) in your brain. Exercise can also help you sleep more soundly. However, don't exercise too close to bedtime because the stimulating release of endorphins might keep you from falling asleep.

## Getting started

There are three aspects to fitness – stamina, strength, and flexibility. Vigorous exercise, such as swimming, jogging, or walking, will improve your stamina and your cardiovascular efficiency. Doctors recommend a minimum of three to four 20-minute sessions per week. Exercise such as lifting weights can improve the strength of your muscles, although it will not improve your cardiovascular fitness. Stretching exercises

## REDUCING THE RISK OF OSTEOPOROSIS

Osteoporosis is a major health problem in the US. Every year, 1.3 million American women over the age of 44 who have osteoporosis fracture one or more bones. Reducing the risk of osteoporosis (and resultant fractures), or postponing its onset, depends on maximizing the levels of bone mass achieved in early adulthood and reducing the rate at which bone is lost from about age 40 onward. The two recommended strategies for achieving these goals are to include an adequate amount of calcium in your diet and to exercise regularly.

◆ Evidence shows that weight-bearing physical activity has a beneficial effect on bone mass. Studies have shown that premenopausal women who exercise regularly have a higher bone mineral content than women who do not exercise. The optimal training program for building bone mineral density has yet to be defined. However, any bone-building exercise regimen needs to incorporate weight-bearing activities such as walking, dancing, or running.

◆ For women who have gone through the menopause, the goal in most cases is to simply retard the rate of bone loss. For this purpose, any level of weight-bearing activity, such as jogging, walking, or stair-climbing (above, right, and below), is helpful.

◆ To get enough exercise to actually increase bone mineral density, postmenopausal women ideally may need to exercise at a relatively intense level 3 days a week for at least 45 minutes. One study included a group of postmenopausal women who did weight-bearing exercises 3 times a week for 50 to 60 minutes. After 9 months, they had an average gain in bone mineral density of 5.2 percent compared to a loss of 1.4 percent in a control group that did not exercise.

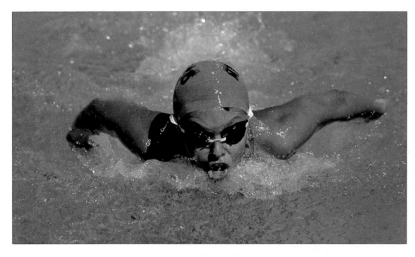

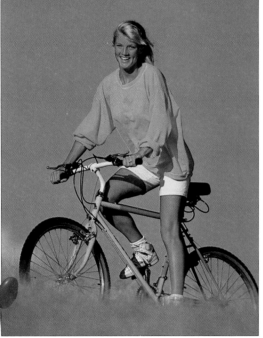

**Losing fat; building muscle**
*Exercise can help you lose weight by increasing the number of calories you burn. Eat a balanced, low-fat diet at the same time. You may not lose weight as soon as you start exercising because exercise increases the bulk of your muscles and muscle weighs more than the same volume of fat. The gain in muscle weight may offset the weight you have lost in fat.*

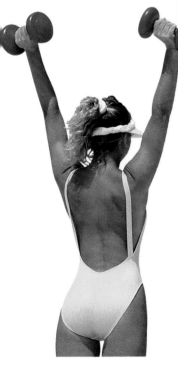

such as those involved in dancing or yoga can improve your flexibility.

Swimming is an excellent form of exercise for women. It improves all three aspects of fitness as well as improving your cardiovascular fitness. It is probably the least physically stressful way to exercise because your weight is supported by water while you swim so pressure on your joints is relieved. Brisk walking is also a good choice for women because it fits easily into everyday life. Walking is an excellent way to embark on a regular fitness program if you have not exercised for a long time.

## ASK YOUR DOCTOR
## DIET AND EXERCISE

**Q** **I am an enthusiastic runner and jog for 3 hours almost every day. Last month I missed my period. Could this have anything to do with the exercise I do?**

**A** It's possible. Women can exercise so much that menstruation stops. This is thought to happen when your percentage of body fat falls below a certain level and your hormone levels are affected, because estrogen is stored in and released from your body fat. You may want to reevaluate your exercise program. Unlike more moderate exercise, vigorous overexercising can contribute to osteoporosis (bone thinning) by causing premature estrogen deficiency.

**Q** **I am 55, slightly overweight, and have not exercised for years. Is it safe for me to jump right into a fitness program?**

**A** You should talk to your doctor first. This recommendation applies to anyone who is overweight, over 35, a smoker, has a family history of heart disease, or has any medical disorder. Your doctor may want to perform a thorough physical examination before discussing the best type of exercise for you.

**Q** **I have heard that weight lifting may help prevent osteoporosis. But will it also build my muscles up too much?**

**A** Weight lifting may help prevent osteoporosis. You are unlikely to build huge muscles. Women lack the male hormone testosterone, and without it even professional women body builders find it difficult to increase the size of their muscles by exercise alone.

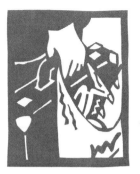

# MANAGING YOUR OPTIONS

**W**OMEN'S WORK can be almost anything today. You can choose traditional roles of homemaker and mother, you can pursue a career, or you can balance several means of personal fulfillment during your lifetime. Sometimes women who are juggling several major obligations experience considerable stress.

## WORK-RELATED STRESS

In addition to stress in your personal life, any of the following job-related factors may increase your stress level:
◆ Work overload
◆ Too much responsibility
◆ Too little control
◆ Unemployment
◆ Boredom
◆ Problems with employers
◆ Unrealistic deadlines
◆ Frequent geographic relocation
◆ Conflict of loyalties
◆ Demotion
◆ Job insecurity

Today a woman has a much wider variety of choices than her ancestors. For many women this freedom has brought new sources of both pressure and satisfaction. Society no longer dictates that a woman stay at home to raise a family while her partner goes to work. A woman may want, and indeed be expected, to combine both work and family. For many women, this new life-style has brought with it considerable stress – both healthy and unhealthy.

## POSITIVE AND NEGATIVE STRESS

Stress is a fact of life. Any form of change, pleasant or not, can be stressful. Examples of positive, life-enhancing stress include a new romance, moving, getting married, getting a promotion, having a baby, and going on a vacation. On the other hand, experiences such as illness, unemployment, bereavement, divorce, debt, or heavy job responsibilities can lead to negative stress. Provided such difficult situations do not occur too frequently or all at once, most women are able to cope with negative stress without long-term ill effects. You can control stress by changing your environment and by changing your expectations (which are often overreactions to your environment). Usually some combination of both works best.

**The working woman**
*More than 60 percent of visits to the doctor in the US are believed to be stress-related, and the most frequent complaints concern work or money anxieties. In the past, men suffered from such problems more than women. However, as the number of women in the work force has increased, women have become as vulnerable as men. Our society is success-oriented, and the pressure to compete and achieve can be stressful.*

## MOTHERHOOD

Raising a family is a full-time occupation and can be highly stressful. Very young children demand constant attention. Anyone whose sleep is regularly disrupted is likely to become exhausted and irritable. Many women do not even realize that they are under stress and feel guilty when they catch themselves losing patience with their children. In addition, the responsibility of rearing children can lead to trouble between parents. The most common problems are uneven division of routine chores and lack of agreement on discipline and education. Stress also may cause sexual difficulties.

When you are at the hub of a busy household , it is easy to undermine yourself by trying to be all things to all people. It can't be done. Concentrate on a few activities that are important and accomplish those.

**The working mother**
*Perhaps the most highly stressed person today is the mother who also works outside the home. She must juggle the demands of her children and her career. She may have little time for relaxation, resulting in long periods of stress. Yet some studies show that working mothers are more content than their nonworking counterparts, perhaps because they find their jobs outside the home rewarding.*

## EFFECTS OF STRESS ON YOUR HEALTH

Everyone has a different level of stress tolerance. Stress can usually be tolerated more easily if it is caused by a temporary problem. Only when a person gets little or no relief from stress can it lead to an inability to cope and a state of continuous anxiety. This long-term stress is usually the result of events over which we feel we have little or no control, such as work problems, illness, bereavement, and financial difficulties. People under stress are more susceptible to illness and are more prone to accidents. Symptoms of stress include:

◆ Headache
◆ Abdominal pain
◆ Chest pain
◆ Sweaty palms
◆ High blood pressure
◆ Menstrual disorders
◆ Inability to concentrate
◆ Indigestion
◆ Dermatitis
◆ Sexual difficulties
◆ Constipation or diarrhea
◆ Asthma
◆ Reliance on alcohol
or other mood-altering drugs

**Long-term stress**
*You may not be aware of the effect of stress on your health until a crisis occurs. If you cannot avoid stress, learn how to recognize warning symptoms when they occur and take steps to prevent the pressures on you from increasing to a level that could harm your health.*

# HOW TO DEAL WITH STRESS

There is no instant way to cope with stress. Long-term use of alcohol or pills does not provide a solution; it creates problems and diminishes your ability to cope with stress. It is much more useful to understand, and respond to, your stressful situation. The first step is to recognize what is causing the stress; then you can decide what you are going to do about it. In many cases, taking almost any action to relieve your stress is a step forward. Remember that many stresses in life involve factors you cannot control. Usually, however, the sources of severe or unavoidable stress tend to change or diminish with time.

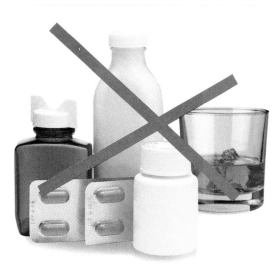

### Work and family
*Be aware of your limitations and be realistic about the demands you make on yourself. Seek the help you need to make life easier. Remember you are just one of the members of an entire household – the other members may need to be reminded to do their share.*

### Demanding children
*The demands of active children can test the patience of an exhausted mother. You may sometimes lose your temper and even feel like hitting your children. If you feel an urge to lash out, go into another room and calm down before you return to deal with the problem. If you feel the tension is building, talk to someone – your partner, a woman who has experienced similar problems, your doctor, or a professional counselor.*

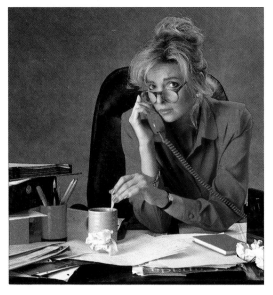

### Work overload
*Talk to your employer about problems you are encountering. He or she should be made aware of the situation; there may be a simple solution. If not, make sure you enjoy yourself outside of work, no matter how busy you are. Try to spend some time each day doing something for yourself. Even a 15-minute bath or a brisk walk can be soothing.*

## Making ends meet

*If you are concerned about your finances, keep a record of your income and all of your expenses and try to find ways to balance the two. If you cannot pay all of your bills, the worst thing you can do is ignore the problem. Contact the people or organizations to whom you owe money without delay; do not ignore any correspondence. An affordable financial counselor can help you organize your spending habits and suggest solutions.*

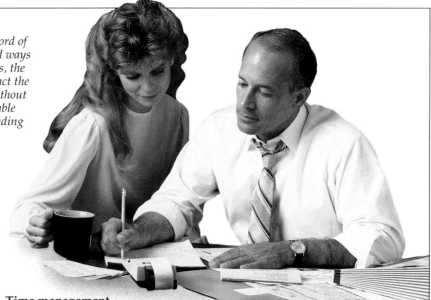

## Time management

*Stress is often caused by mismanagement of time. Make a list each day of everything you need to do, assign priorities, and complete your tasks in order of importance. This type of system ensures that you always end each day with some sense of achievement.*

## Exercise

*Regular exercise can relax you and counteract stress as well as encourage the physical tiredness to help you sleep well. Choose a form of exercise that you enjoy and will want to do regularly – for example, swim, jog, play tennis, or walk. Try to build exercise into your daily schedule – for instance, by walking to the store or to the train. Yoga may also help; it requires no special equipment, it can be practiced safely at all ages, it promotes suppleness, and it is a relaxation technique.*

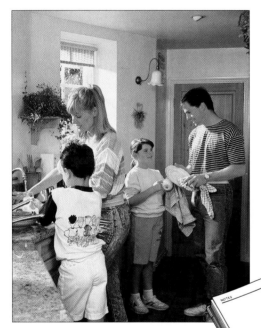

## Routine chores

*Decide with your partner how the two of you can share the household responsibilities. Ask your children to help as well. Though they may be reluctant at first, most children actually begin to enjoy their new responsibilities. A chart may help everyone keep track of his or her job.*

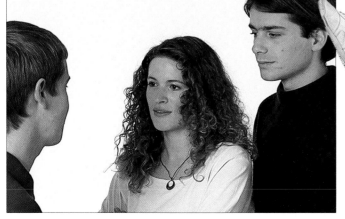

## Marital problems

*One in two marriages in the US ends in divorce. If your relationship is no longer successful, do not assume that it is your fault or place all the blame on your partner. You may benefit from counseling. However, you may finally decide that divorce is your only option. While divorce is a traumatic experience, it can offer release from a stressful life with an incompatible partner and offer hope for the future.*

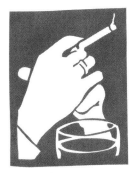

# UNDERSTANDING HEALTH HAZARDS

YOU DO ALL THE RIGHT THINGS to take care of your body – you exercise regularly, eat a healthy diet, and successfully manage the stresses in your life. What more can you do? Do no harm. You can avoid those activities and hazards in your environment that pose a definite threat to your health and well-being.

Smoking, drinking too much alcohol, misusing other drugs, or having unprotected sexual intercourse can increase your risk of a number of diseases and health problems. Fortunately, these factors are entirely within your control.

## SHORT-TERM EFFECTS OF SMOKING

Although the long-term ill effects of smoking are well publicized, the short-term effects are perhaps less well understood.

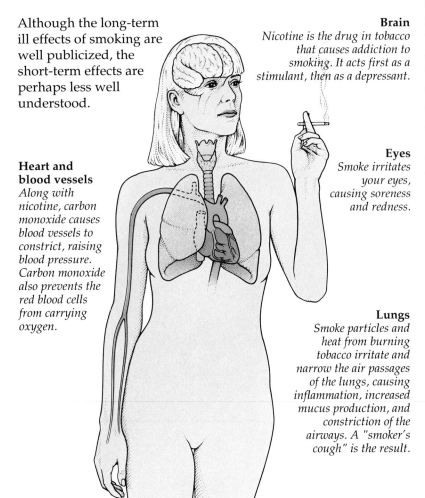

**Brain**
*Nicotine is the drug in tobacco that causes addiction to smoking. It acts first as a stimulant, then as a depressant.*

**Heart and blood vessels**
*Along with nicotine, carbon monoxide causes blood vessels to constrict, raising blood pressure. Carbon monoxide also prevents the red blood cells from carrying oxygen.*

**Eyes**
*Smoke irritates your eyes, causing soreness and redness.*

**Lungs**
*Smoke particles and heat from burning tobacco irritate and narrow the air passages of the lungs, causing inflammation, increased mucus production, and constriction of the airways. A "smoker's cough" is the result.*

## SMOKING

Under the age of 65, smokers have a death rate double that of nonsmokers. Tobacco smoking is the main cause of lung cancer; it is a significant factor in deaths from chronic bronchitis, emphysema, and heart disease; and it is an important cause of cancers of the mouth, tongue, lips, larynx, esophagus, bladder, and cervix. An increase in the number of women smokers has resulted in an increase in female mortality from lung cancer – the female death rate is three times as high as it was 35 years ago. The risk of smoking-related disease starts to diminish as soon as you quit, and the longer you abstain, the less likely you are to die of a disease caused by smoking.

### Smoking and pregnancy

Smoking during pregnancy can seriously affect a fetus's development. Every cigarette a pregnant woman smokes supplies nicotine, tar, and carbon monoxide that cross the placenta to the fetus's bloodstream. The carbon monoxide reduces the ability of the fetus's red blood cells to take up oxygen, depriving the fetus of a vital substance. The fetus's rate of metabolism is reduced and fetal development and rate of growth is inhibited. Compared to nonsmokers' babies, babies of smokers have a low birth weight, their resistance to disease is low, and their ability to breathe is impaired.

## ALCOHOL

In small quantities, alcohol may not appear to have any harmful effects on the body. However, alcohol is a drug, and significant numbers of people who drink alcohol become addicted to it. Even moderate amounts of alcohol can damage your body. Regular, heavy drinking that may not cause drunkenness or social embarrassment can nevertheless seriously damage your liver, heart, brain, and other organs. In developed countries, the number of women drinkers has greatly increased in recent years. Ounce for ounce, alcohol is more dangerous to women than men because of the difference between the two sexes in stomach enzymes that metabolize alcohol. In some recent studies, more alcohol reached women's bloodstreams because they were less able than men to break down alcohol in their stomachs. Alcohol is a significant factor in automobile accidents as well as domestic violence, child abuse, and other types of crimes that involve both men and women.

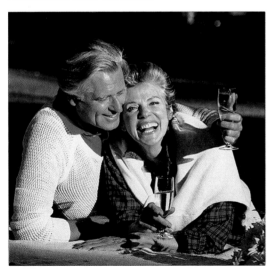

**Drink for drink**
*Some studies show that a woman's drinking pattern often correlates with her male partner's drinking pattern. A woman usually matches her partner drink for drink. Yet, to reach a given blood alcohol level, a woman needs to consume only about half of what a man does, in part because she has significantly less of certain stomach enzymes that break down alcohol.*

## HOW ALCOHOL AFFECTS YOUR BODY

In addition to altering your mood, alcohol has a range of other effects on your body. High intake of alcoholic beverages increases the risk of cancers of the mouth, throat, larynx, and esophagus.

**Brain**
*Alcohol acts as a depressant on the brain, decreasing its activity, and reducing anxiety, tension, and inhibition. In small amounts, it can provide a feeling of confidence and relaxation. However, the longer you continue to drink, the more your concentration and judgment are impaired. If you drink an excessive amount, the effects can range from lack of coordination to unconsciousness.*

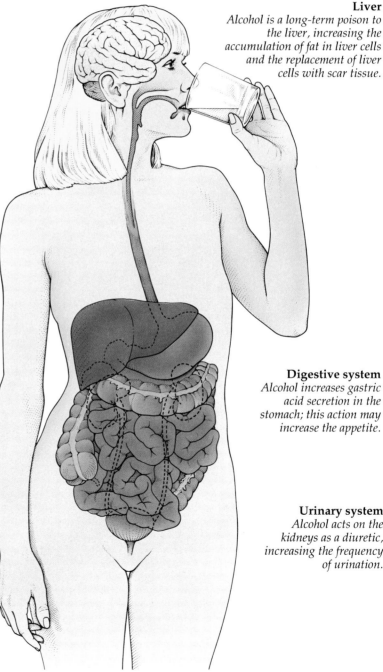

**Liver**
*Alcohol is a long-term poison to the liver, increasing the accumulation of fat in liver cells and the replacement of liver cells with scar tissue.*

**Digestive system**
*Alcohol increases gastric acid secretion in the stomach; this action may increase the appetite.*

**Urinary system**
*Alcohol acts on the kidneys as a diuretic, increasing the frequency of urination.*

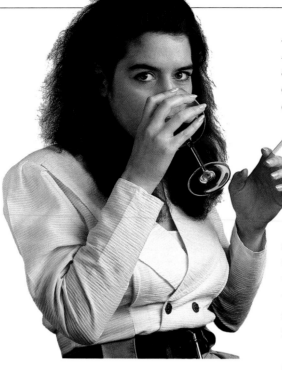

**Recognizing alcohol addiction**
*Alcoholism may be associated with behavioral changes such as aggressiveness, irritability, neglect of food intake and personal appearance, and long periods of drunkenness. Physical symptoms include nausea, vomiting and shaking in the morning, abdominal pain, weakness of the arms and legs, confusion, poor memory, and incontinence.*

# Alcohol addiction

Alcohol addiction (alcoholism) is characterized by habitual, compulsive consumption of alcohol and the development of withdrawal symptoms when drinking is suddenly stopped. For many women, the transition from social drinking to addiction is so gradual they don't notice until addiction is well established. The prevalence of alcoholism among American women has increased slightly in recent years. In the population as a whole, estimates indicate that three in 50 people in the US are addicted to alcohol. Genetic predisposition to alcoholism may play a role, although it has not been proved conclusively.

Long-term heavy use of alcohol can cause serious disorders, including cancers of the esophagus, liver, and mouth; alcoholic hepatitis and cirrhosis; nervous system degeneration; and heart and circulatory disorders. Alcohol can also intensify osteoporosis in women who smoke and drink.

## SEXUAL PRACTICES

Women today are strongly advised not to have unprotected sexual intercourse with any new partners, particularly if they are unsure of the person's sexual history. Potential hazards include sexual transmission of the human immunodeficiency virus (HIV), which causes AIDS, or other sexually transmitted diseases (STDs) such as genital herpes, chlamydial infection of the uterus or fallopian tubes, human papillomavirus, syphilis, or gonorrhea.

The rate of heterosexual transmission of HIV varies considerably throughout the world. By the end of 1988, the US Centers for Disease Control reported 3,570 cases of AIDS transmitted by heterosexuals in the US. The risk of contracting HIV is increased if you have any form of genital ulceration, which may result from irritation or infection. The number of new cases of AIDS in women of reproductive age continues to increase. If current trends continue, AIDS will become one of the leading causes of death among women of childbearing age.

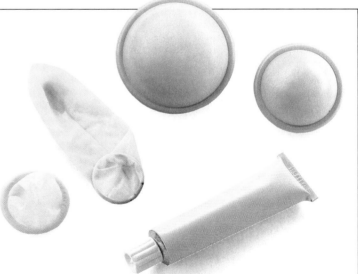

**Barrier methods**
*A condom offers the most effective protection against most sexually transmitted diseases (STDs) provided your male partner puts it on his penis before it touches your genital area. Condoms should be used with spermicides, especially those containing nonoxynol 9, which provides some protection against HIV. Contraceptive diaphragms can protect against STDs that affect the cervix and reproductive organs, but they do not protect against other STDs as effectively as the condom does.*

## DRUG USE AND PREGNANCY

If you have been using any drugs – including alcohol, tobacco, and prescription and over-the-counter medications – and you become pregnant, see your doctor immediately. If you are planning to become pregnant, it is even better to talk to your doctor about any drugs you may be taking before conceiving. Use of some drugs increases the risk of miscarriage and birth defects in the early months of pregnancy and of premature labor in the later stages. If you need to take drugs for a medical reason after your baby is born, consult your doctor about the pros and cons of breast-feeding; many drugs can be passed on to your baby.

### Supervised withdrawal

*If you have been taking opiates, barbiturates, tranquilizers, or any sedative-type drugs and you become pregnant, it is important to stop taking the drugs gradually to avoid danger to the fetus. Most doctors recommend that you follow a monitored withdrawal program in which a safer drug at a lower dosage is substituted, to reduce the risk to the fetus.*

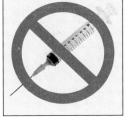

### DRUG ABUSE

Drug abuse is defined as any use of drugs that causes physical, psychological, economic, legal, or social harm to the user or to people affected by the user's behavior. Illegal drugs of abuse include marijuana, cocaine, LSD, heroin, and morphine. Legal drugs that are commonly abused are alcohol, tobacco, benzodiazepines (anti-anxiety drugs), synthetic narcotics, and amphetamines.

## DRUGS OF ABUSE

In most developed countries, alcohol and tobacco are categorized as legal drugs, while substances such as marijuana, heroin, and cocaine are categorized as illegal. Prescription drugs can also be abused; for example, tranquilizers and stimulants are often sold illegally. Every year in the US, many fatalities occur as a direct result of the misuse of psychoactive drugs such as those prescribed to treat depression and anxiety.

## What can drug abuse do?

Drug abuse can cause many disorders, including menstrual irregularities and reduced fertility, serious disorders of the neuromuscular system, impaired concentration, drowsiness, and coma. However, drug abuse is not only potentially devastating to your physical health, it can also seriously damage your emotional well-being and relationships. Some female addicts turn to prostitution to support their habits. This increases their risk of acquiring a sexually trans-mitted disease, as well as exposing them to the risk of abuse. Drug and alcohol use are implicated in the majority of child-abuse and spouse-abuse incidents as well as triggering many other violent crimes such as murder and armed robbery. In addition, drug use is the cause of many motor vehicle and boating accidents as well as accidents in the home.

### Women and drugs

*About 70 percent of the mood-altering drugs (such as benzodiazepines, used to treat anxiety) prescribed every year are for women. Benzodiazepines and other tranquilizers should be used only temporarily at a time of crisis or when severe anxiety interferes with your sleep. Psychotherapy, sometimes in combination with antidepressants, is a better solution for anxiety than tranquilizers.*

# CHAPTER THREE

# SEX AND CONTRACEPTION

INTRODUCTION

WOMEN'S SEXUAL
EXPERIENCE

CONTRACEPTION

TODAY, WOMEN in the US are more able to express their sexuality than at any previous time. This freedom partly results from the changing role of women in society and changing attitudes toward sex. It is also, in large part, the result of a major development – the availability of the contraceptive pill and several other effective birth-control methods. With this sexual freedom, women are confronted with new responsibilities and decisions to make about their sexual and reproductive lives. In the early 1980s, doctors became concerned that women taking the contraceptive pill might be at increased risk of blood clotting abnormalities and certain types of cancer. However, most doctors now believe that many of the potentially harmful side effects caused by early types of contraceptive pills were related to the comparatively large doses of hormones that the pills contained. The low-dose versions available today are thought to be much safer. Furthermore, the risk of the pill causing breast and cervical cancers is small and the pill actually provides protection against ovarian and uterine cancers.

A woman's sexual function is by no means restricted to her reproductive system. Her general health is an important aspect of her sexual life. A woman's sexuality also en-

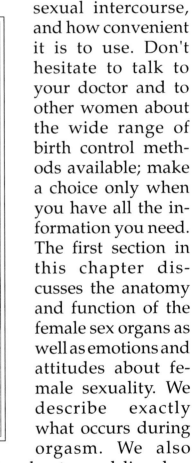

compasses her emotions and feelings throughout every stage in her life – puberty, pregnancy and childbirth, menopause, and her later years. Choosing an appropriate method of contraception is, for most American women, an important consideration. The method of contraception that a woman uses should depend not only on its effectiveness but on whether it affects her or her partner's health, how much it interferes with sexual intercourse, and how convenient it is to use. Don't hesitate to talk to your doctor and to other women about the wide range of birth control methods available; make a choice only when you have all the information you need. The first section in this chapter discusses the anatomy and function of the female sex organs as well as emotions and attitudes about female sexuality. We describe exactly what occurs during orgasm. We also provide information about sexual disorders to help you recognize and overcome them. The second section in this chapter explains new and future contraceptive choices. It reviews the methods of birth control now available in the US, including barrier methods, the contraceptive pill, intrauterine devices, hormonal implants, and sterilization. Future options, such as contraceptive vaccines, are also discussed.

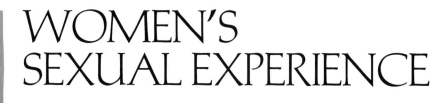

# WOMEN'S SEXUAL EXPERIENCE

A WOMAN'S SEXUAL LIFE is marked by physical and emotional change, such as the onset of menstruation, falling in love, her first experience of sexual intercourse, pregnancy and childbirth, and the menopause. How she experiences and responds to each of these changes has a profound effect on her sexuality.

As she becomes sexually mature, a young woman experiences many physical changes, all of which have a strong influence on her sexual awareness and self-confidence. Every woman should get to know her body and become familiar with her sexual organs in order to better understand their function. Getting to know your physical self can also help you overcome any embarrassment you may associate with these intimate parts of your body.

## THE EXTERNAL SEX ORGANS

The external, visible structures of a woman's reproductive system are collectively known as the vulva. The vulva is erogenous (sexually sensitive) and highly responsive to touch; it also protects the vaginal and urethral openings.

### The hymen
*The hymen is a thin layer of tissue that partially or completely covers the entrance to the vagina in childhood. An intact hymen usually allows a small speculum (medical examining device) or tampon to be inserted. Vigorous physical activity or sexual intercourse may stretch or tear the hymen. This process may or may not be painful or cause bleeding. Rarely, if there is no opening for menstruation or if the hymen is too strong and resistant to allow intercourse, the tissue may require surgical incision.*

### The mons pubis
*The mons pubis is the curved, sloping area of tissue in front of the genitals that becomes covered with hair after puberty. The hard ridge of the pubic bone, which forms the front of the pelvis, lies at the bottom of the mons pubis.*

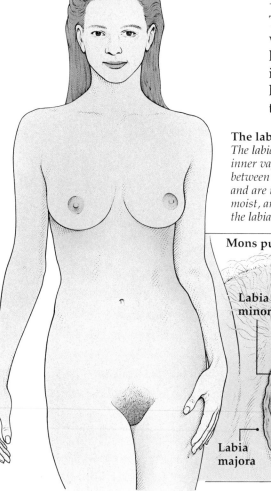

### The labia minora
*The labia minora are the inner vaginal lips. They lie between the labia majora and are more pink, smooth, moist, and delicate than the labia majora.*

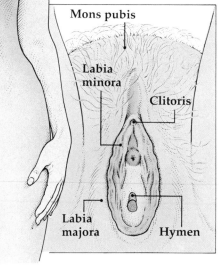

Mons pubis

Labia minora

Clitoris

Labia majora

Hymen

### The labia majora
*The labia majora are the two external lips that form the outermost part of the vulva. The lips usually lie close together, protecting the other genital organs. The labia majora are thick, fleshy, and irregularly formed, and they vary widely in color and shape.*

### The clitoris
*The clitoris lies at the front of the vagina, between the folds of the labia. The clitoris is rich in nerve endings and, for most women, it is the most sensitive part of the genitalia. During sexual excitement, the small erectile tip of the clitoris, usually hidden from view and protected by a thick hood of skin, becomes more prominent.*

# THE INTERNAL SEX ORGANS

Your internal sex organs include your uterus and cervix, fallopian tubes, and ovaries. They are connected to the outside of your body by the vagina. The internal structures are supported by ligaments and muscles that hold them securely in place, while allowing for the movement and growth that is essential during the stages of pregnancy.

**The fallopian tubes**
*The fallopian tubes extend from the uterus to each of the two ovaries. Each funnel-shaped tube is about 3 inches long; the narrow end opens into the uterus, and the free, expanded end lies close to the ovary. Each month, one of these tubes actively propels an unfertilized or fertilized egg into the uterus.*

**The uterus**
*The uterus is shaped like an upside-down pear. It is about 3½ inches long and 2½ inches wide at its widest point, but expands to 30 times this size during pregnancy. The walls of the uterus consist of a network of thick, flexible muscle fibers.*

**The ovaries**
*The ovaries are a pair of almond-shaped glands situated on either side of the uterus, immediately below the openings of the fallopian tubes. Each ovary is about 1¼ inches long and ¾ inch wide and contains multiple cavities, called follicles, in which ova (eggs) develop. In addition to producing eggs, the ovaries produce the female sex hormones estrogen and progesterone.*

Ovary

Fallopian tube

Uterus

Bladder

Cervix

Vagina

Urethra

**The urethra**
*The bladder lies in front of the upper half of the vagina; the tube leading from the bladder to the outside of the body is called the urethra. Compared to a man's urethra, a woman's urethra is more easily exposed to and contaminated by bacteria, such as those encountered during intercourse or contained in fecal matter. These bacteria can enter and infect the bladder.*

**The vagina**
*The vagina, which is about 4 inches long, is the passage leading from the uterus to the outside of the body. The vagina secretes a moist fluid that carries organisms with it when it leaves the body and facilitates sexual intercourse.*

**The cervix**
*The cervix is a cylindrical organ that lies at the lowest part of the uterus, projecting into the vagina. The cervix is soft and has some muscle. After puberty it secretes mucus. It has a dimplelike opening in its center (called the cervical os) that allows for the passage of menstrual blood and semen and for childbirth. Cervical mucus changes in color and consistency at different times of the menstrual cycle. At ovulation, the cervical os opens and the mucus becomes thinner and more favorable to the transportation of sperm.*

# WHAT HAPPENS DURING ORGASM?

Orgasm is the extremely pleasurable, spontaneous reflex action of the body that releases the physical tension built up during sexual stimulation. A sequence of physiological changes leads to orgasm. This sequence has four stages – arousal, plateau, climax, and resolution. On the average, a woman reaches orgasm 14 minutes after initial arousal.

### Plateau

*The plateau is the second stage of the process that leads to orgasm; it occurs just before the climax. It is basically an intensification of the arousal stage. The woman's heart rate and blood pressure increase further, and her breathing remains heavy. Slight enlargement of her breasts, areolae, and nipples continues, and she may begin to make involuntary, spasmodic movements as muscular tension increases. The vulva becomes redder, and the inner part of the vagina opens and widens. The clitoris appears to retract within the hood as the hood enlarges.*

**PLATEAU PHASE OF EXCITEMENT**

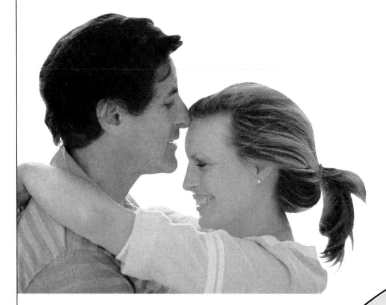

**Uterus**

**Bladder**

**Clitoris**

**Vagina**

**INITIAL AROUSAL**

**UNAROUSED STATE**

### Arousal

*Arousal, or excitement, is the first stage in the process that leads to orgasm; it may last a few minutes to several hours. Arousal involves a number of physical changes. The breasts swell slightly and become more sensitive. The nipples become firm and erect and the areolae (the dark areas around the nipples) swell. Heart rate increases, blood pressure rises, and breathing becomes heavier. A slight increase in the surface temperature of the body, with flushing and mottling of the skin, may occur. A woman may feel hot and start to sweat, particularly in the armpits and around the vulva. This sweat often carries powerful hormonelike stimulants called pheromones, the odor of which may intensify arousal. The woman's eyes may look darker, as the pupil enlarges.*

### PROBLEMS WITH ORGASM

Anorgasmia is the medical term for difficulty reaching orgasm. In women, anorgasmia is the largest category of sexual dysfunction, accounting for a high percentage of women who seek sex therapy. There are several categories of anorgasmia, including women who have never had an orgasm, women who regularly had orgasms at one time but no longer do, and women who experience orgasm only under certain circumstances (for example, when they masturbate). However, a woman who only occasionally achieves orgasm should be considered to have a dysfunction only if the situation causes her distress or dissatisfaction. Most women do not reach orgasm during intercourse.

## Climax

*If stimulation continues, the plateau stage advances into the climax, or orgasm. The climax is a series of contractions centered in the muscles surrounding the vagina and perineum (the area between the vulva and anus), but the contractions may also be felt in other areas of the body such as the uterus, stomach, anus, and legs. Each contraction lasts about $1/8$ second and is very quickly followed by the next one. Blood pressure, heart rate, and breathing rate reach their peak.*

## Multiple orgasm

*Unlike men, who need a period of rest before they can ejaculate a second time, women can climax again and again (so-called multiple orgasm) provided that stimulation does not stop. Not all women experience multiple orgasm.*

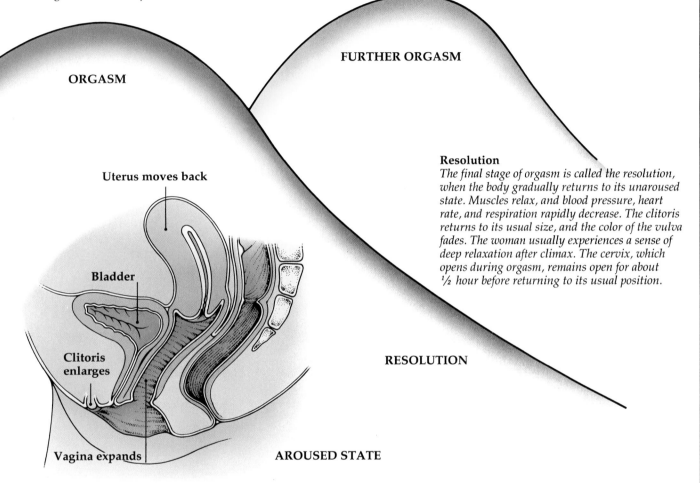

**FURTHER ORGASM**

**ORGASM**

## Resolution

*The final stage of orgasm is called the resolution, when the body gradually returns to its unaroused state. Muscles relax, and blood pressure, heart rate, and respiration rapidly decrease. The clitoris returns to its usual size, and the color of the vulva fades. The woman usually experiences a sense of deep relaxation after climax. The cervix, which opens during orgasm, remains open for about $1/2$ hour before returning to its usual position.*

**Uterus moves back**

**Bladder**

**Clitoris enlarges**

**RESOLUTION**

**Vagina expands**

**AROUSED STATE**

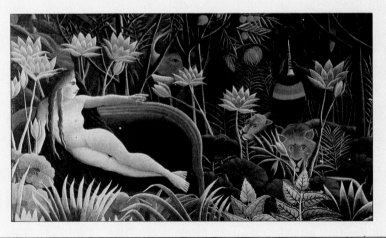

## Treatment of anorgasmia

*The origins of anorgasmia are psychological in most cases, although many anorgasmic women are emotionally healthy and there is a definite reason for their problem. In only 5 percent of cases is anorgasmia caused by a physical condition. Common treatment techniques for anorgasmia include encouraging a woman to explore her body and sexual response, dealing with any anxiety about performance, improving communication between the woman and her partner, and reducing her sexual inhibitions.*

# SEXUAL RHYTHMS

Many women experience two peaks of sexual desire during each menstrual cycle (see chart below). One occurs just before (or, less commonly, during) menstruation. The other, usually less intense, occurs at the time of ovulation. "Biological logic" may underlie the latter peak in desire because, at midcycle, around the time of ovulation, a woman is most likely to conceive. In contrast, the sexual peak around the time of menstruation seems not to have any purpose but perhaps relates to the swelling of the clitoris that occurs because of generalized water retention. A woman who is taking the contraceptive pill may respond sexually at about the same level throughout her cycle because of the constant levels of synthetic hormones in her system. A woman who is breast-feeding may experience arousal as a result of the baby's sucking. Some breast-feeding women neither ovulate nor menstruate so they may not notice any variation. Others produce a very high level of prolactin, a hormone that stimulates milk secretion and also can inhibit sexual desire. It is helpful to be aware of your personal sexual rhythm and its fluctuations so that you can understand and enjoy your body. If you are relying on abstinence from intercourse during your fertile time as your means of contraception, you must be aware that your sexual desire may peak just when intercourse presents the greatest likelihood of pregnancy. This is one of the reasons natural family planning (see page 70) is unreliable.

**Lesbianism and bisexuality**
*Some women are sexually and emotionally attracted to other women, and some are attracted to both sexes. These are considered variations in sexual orientation and are not disorders. A woman who is distressed about her sexual orientation may seek counseling to resolve emotional problems. The causes of sexual orientation are not known. Genetic, hormonal, and developmental factors probably act in concert and the importance of each factor varies among individuals. Sexual orientation is determined very early in life.*

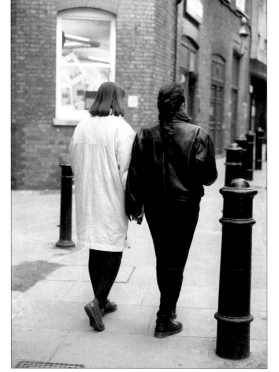

# ORAL SEX

Oral sex is stimulation by mouth of the male genitals (fellatio) or the female genitals (cunnilingus). Oral sex has been accepted and practiced for centuries in nearly all cultures. Most couples enjoy both forms of oral sex but some women and men still feel hesitant. Sometimes it helps to read about sexual techniques with your partner – shared reading can be a valuable introduction to shared experience. However, what you and your partner choose to include in or exclude

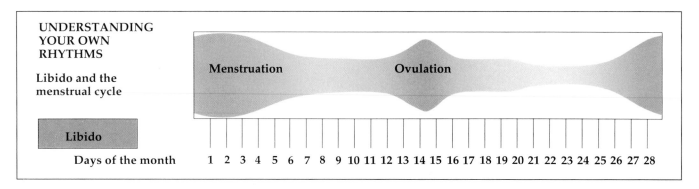

**UNDERSTANDING YOUR OWN RHYTHMS**

**Libido and the menstrual cycle**

Menstruation    Ovulation

Libido

Days of the month    1  2  3  4  5  6  7  8  9  10  11  12  13  14  15  16  17  18  19  20  21  22  23  24  25  26  27  28

from your sexual practices is your decision; neither of you should feel under pressure to do anything you do not want to do. Differences in sexual preferences are neither good nor bad. You may negotiate with your partner and compromise if necessary so that each of your needs can be met.

# SEXUAL DISORDERS

Women seek professional help as often as men do to deal with sexual problems. Some sexual disorders have psychological origins and are the result of sexual ignorance, inhibitions, religious beliefs, or problems in the relationship between partners. Other sexual disorders have a physical cause such as an intact hymen or thinning or inflammation of the vaginal lining after menopause.

### Sexual inhibitions
*Inhibitions are negative feelings that interfere with a person's enjoyment of sex and make it difficult for him or her to respond sexually. Many sexual inhibitions are rooted in outdated ideas about appropriate sexual behavior for women and men. Inhibitions also serve to protect against unwanted consequences of sex such as pregnancy, sexually transmitted diseases, or feelings of exploitation or rejection. Building trust in a relationship reduces these risks. Most contemporary women have overcome sexual inhibition on an intellectual level but may still find it difficult to express themselves freely in a sexual way. Women who do not enjoy sex may find help in counseling.*

## MASTURBATION
Contrary to some earlier beliefs, masturbation is not abnormal. Most women masturbate. Early in life, both boys and girls discover, as part of the normal healthy process of self-exploration, that touching their genitals brings them great pleasure. Many of them go on to discover how to achieve orgasm. For both sexes, this self-discovery is a vital part of sexual development. Most people need to learn to enjoy their own bodies before experiencing satisfying sexual exchange with another person.

## LACK OF SEXUAL DESIRE

A loss of sexual desire and lack of interest in sexual activity is not unusual. There are many possible reasons for these feelings. For some women, the desire for sex fluctuates with the opportunity for partnership and intercourse. A gradual loss of interest sometimes occurs between long-term partners. A number of factors (including those listed below) can block, prevent, or even destroy sexual desire. In most cases, a woman can restore her sexual desire when the factors are resolved. Sexual desire can be reduced by:

◆ Conflict or anger in a relationship
◆ Fatigue
◆ Grief or other type of loss
◆ Stress
◆ Illness or disability
◆ Depression or anxiety
◆ Excessive alcohol consumption or other drug use
◆ Overeating
◆ Use of some medications
◆ Recent childbirth
◆ Menopausal changes

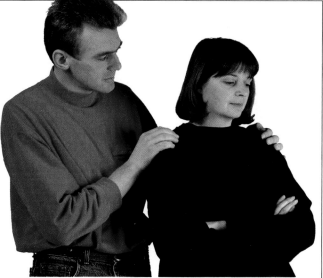

### Sex drive
*A mutual desire for sex helps to nurture a relationship. Try not to be concerned if your partner has a higher or lower sex drive than you. If your partner's libido is lower than yours, keep in mind that it may simply be a difference and no one is to blame. You can compensate with mutual stimulation or masturbation. Sexual intensity is not the only measure of satisfaction; closeness and affection are more important than how often you have sex.*

## Vaginismus

Vaginismus is a painful spasm of the circular muscles of the lower third of the vagina that makes intercourse difficult, uncomfortable, or impossible. A woman who suffers from vaginismus also may or may not be able to tolerate an internal pelvic medical examination or may not be able to insert a tampon.

Vaginismus usually (although not always) occurs as the result of a sexually repressive upbringing or an abusive sexual experience such as rape or childhood sexual abuse. The woman's fear causes her vaginal muscles to tense up as a protective mechanism against anticipated pain from intercourse. The vaginal muscles can become conditioned to respond in this way and may tense up as an automatic or reflex response to any suggestion of sexual contact even with the most gentle, loving partner.

## PAIN DURING INTERCOURSE

Dyspareunia is the medical term for pain at the entrance to or deeper within the vagina experienced during sexual intercourse. If you experience any unusual pain during intercourse, make an ap-

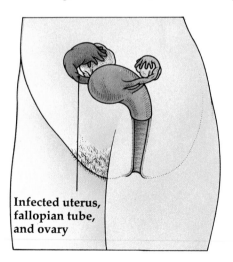

**Pelvic inflammatory disease**
*Pelvic inflammatory disease, in which the reproductive organs become inflamed and tender, is a common cause of deep dyspareunia.*

Infected uterus, fallopian tube, and ovary

**Treatment for vaginismus**
*If you think you may have vaginismus, talk to your doctor. He or she may recommend a self-help program or you may be referred to a psychotherapist. A program of vaginal relaxation exercises, in which the woman practices stretching her vaginal opening in a nonthreatening situation, can help alleviate vaginismus. Later, a trusted sexual partner can help with these exercises. A combination of behavior modification and psychotherapy has a high rate of success.*

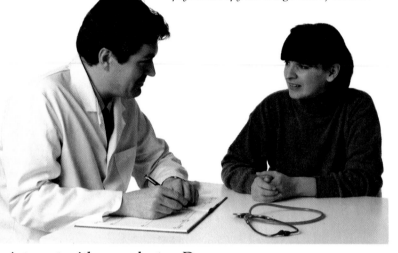

pointment with your doctor. Dyspareunia may be caused by several physical and psychological factors but it should always be fully investigated.

## Superficial dyspareunia

Superficial dyspareunia is pain felt at the entrance to the vagina. It can be caused by vaginal inflammation, infection, or insufficient vaginal lubrication. A woman may not lubricate enough if she is not fully sexually aroused, if she has gone through the menopause, or if she has recently given birth to a baby.

## Deep dyspareunia

Deep dyspareunia is pain deep in the vagina or lower part of the abdomen. It may originate from a pelvic infection such as pelvic inflammatory disease, in which the reproductive organs become inflamed and tender (left). A second possible cause is endometriosis, a condition in which tissue similar to the tissue in the lining of the uterus attaches to and grows in inappropriate places such as the ovaries or pelvic lining. A gynecological checkup is essential.

**PSYCHOLOGICAL CAUSES OF DYSPAREUNIA**

A woman who has experienced childhood sexual abuse or rape may have dyspareunia. In some cases, fear of pregnancy, severe conflict in a relationship, or personal stress may cause dyspareunia. A thorough evaluation for both physical and psychological causes of dyspareunia is recommended for any woman with this problem. Psychotherapy may help a woman work through psychological causes for her condition or may help her cope with problems caused by a chronic disease such as endometriosis.

# CASE HISTORY
# PAINFUL INTERCOURSE

FOR SEVERAL WEEKS, **Linda avoided having intercourse with her husband Tom because she found it painful. They had always enjoyed a satisfying sexual relationship and she knew of no reason for her discomfort. Because of the pain and because she missed sexual intimacy with her husband, Linda made an appointment to see her doctor about the problem.**

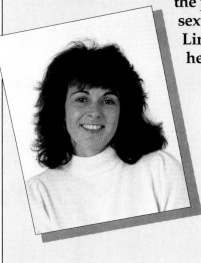

**PERSONAL DETAILS**
**Name** Linda Walker
**Age** 34
**Occupation** Seamstress
**Family** Parents are well.
Linda has two healthy children.

## THE DIAGNOSIS

The results of the tests confirm that Linda has VAGINITIS (inflammation of the vagina). Her vaginitis is caused by infection with the fungus *Candida albicans*. Linda is prescribed a vaginal cream containing an antifungal agent. The doctor reassures Linda that vaginal infection is a common complication of even short courses of antibiotic therapy because the antibiotic destroys the normal protective vaginal bacteria that usually control growth of fungus. Linda's infection has not come from any other source. The doctor advises Linda to avoid intercourse for a week and to come back if her symptoms get worse or do not improve.

## THE OUTCOME

After completing her course of medication, Linda has no symptoms of fungal infection. With the symptoms gone, her sexual desire returns and intercourse is no longer painful, so she does not need to see her doctor again. She and her husband resume their active sex life.

## MEDICAL BACKGROUND

Linda's pregnancies were both well planned and uncomplicated. She has never had a sexually transmitted disease. Two months ago Linda contracted a relatively minor chest infection for which she was prescribed a 2-week course of antibiotics.

## THE CONSULTATION

Linda tells her doctor that she and Tom have always enjoyed sex together, but that lately she has found it painful. As Linda talks, her doctor concludes that there is no emotional reason for her symptoms. Linda says she has felt run-down since her illness. Questioning her further, Linda's doctor learns that her pain occurs during penetration and began about a week after she started taking antibiotics. When the doctor performs a gynecological examination, she finds that the entrance to Linda's vagina is very inflamed, with a few white patches on the inner vaginal walls and on the cervix. She takes a series of vaginal swabs that she will evaluate under a microscope in her office laboratory.

**Vaginitis**
*The photograph above (magnified 400 times) shows cells of* Candida albicans, *the fungus responsible for Linda's vaginitis.*

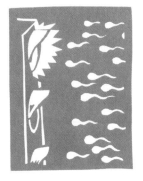

# CONTRACEPTION

**F**OR THOUSANDS OF YEARS, women have been using whatever contraceptive methods were available to them. The Bible refers to coitus interruptus, and ancient Egyptian records describe the use of honey douches and spermicidal concoctions made of crocodile dung. The first rubber condom appeared in 1842. However, it was the development of the combined contraceptive pill in 1960 that truly revolutionized contraceptive practices.

In contrast to the diaphragm, the condom, and withdrawal, all of which require effort at the time of intercourse, the contraceptive pill separates the act of intercourse from the process of contraception. It offers a woman a reliable form of birth control that does not require cooperation from her partner.

## CONTRACEPTION: A TYPICAL LIFE HISTORY

## TYPES OF CONTRACEPTION

There are many types of contraception available today and each type interferes with the process of reproduction in a different way. A contraceptive may prevent sperm from entering the uterus (barrier methods, coitus interruptus, and vasectomy); kill sperm before they

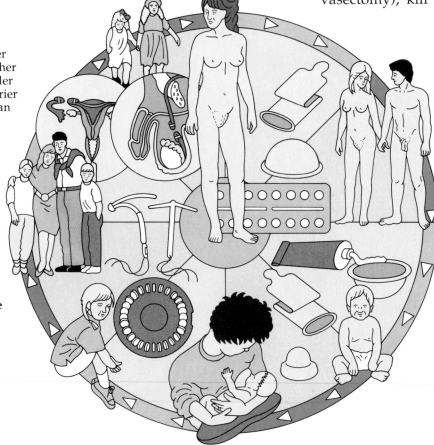

**After completing** her family, a woman or her husband may consider sterilization or a barrier method or the woman may use an IUD.

**If more children are planned**, the combined pill can help regulate menstrual cycles and prevent conception between pregnancies.

**A woman** who is not in an established relationship can use a barrier method for protection against AIDS and other sexually transmitted diseases as well as to prevent pregnancy. She also may wish to take the combined contraceptive pill.

**In a marriage** or an established relationship, a woman may use only the pill. If she wants to have a baby, she may choose to use only a barrier method for about 3 months before trying to conceive.

**If a woman is breast-feeding,** use of a barrier method or the minipill is recommended.

reach the egg (spermicides and intrauterine devices); block sperm from reaching the egg via the fallopian tubes (tubal ligation); block the release of a mature egg (the combined oral contraceptive pill); stop a fertilized egg from implanting in the lining of the uterus (a secondary action of intrauterine devices and the primary action of the progestin-only contraceptive pill, also called the mini-pill); or limit intercourse to infertile times of the month (periodic abstinence).

## Choosing your method of contraception

It is well worth your time to research the many different types of contraception available before deciding which method is best for you. One major reason for contraceptive failure is a lack of understanding of the method being used. Your doctor can help answer questions about the risks and benefits of each kind.

You and your partner need to consider options in terms of effectiveness, safety, convenience, and sexual satisfaction. Apart from sexual abstinence, the combined pill is the most effective

### HOW SUCCESSFUL ARE DIFFERENT METHODS OF CONTRACEPTION?

**Number of pregnancies per 100 women who use the method for 1 year**

| Method | If used perfectly | If not used perfectly |
|---|---|---|
| Combined pill | Less than 1 | 2 |
| Condom used with contraceptive foam | Less than 1 | 5 |
| Contraceptive foams, creams, suppositories, and sponges | 5 to 15 | 15 to 30 |
| Diaphragm used with contraceptive cream or jelly | 2 | 10 |
| Implant | Less than 0.5 | — |
| Injection | Less than 2 | — |
| IUD | 2 | 4 |
| Minipill | Less than 1 | 4 |
| Natural methods | 2 to 20 | 20 to 30 |
| Sterilization | Less than 2 out of 1,000 | — |
| Withdrawal | 5 | 20 |

## RISK OF DEATH FROM CONTRACEPTIVE PILL USAGE AND FROM CHILDBIRTH

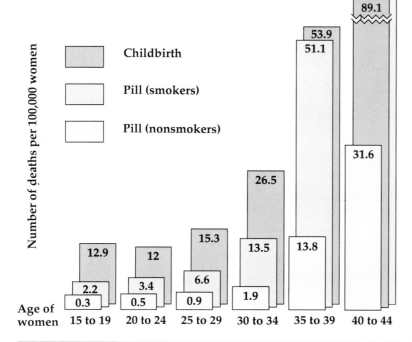

method of contraception. However, unlike the condom, it does not protect against sexually transmitted diseases. Many women prefer sterilization or nonhormonal contraceptives such as IUDs or diaphragms. Some may have limited choices for medical reasons. For example, smokers over 35 should not use oral contraceptives because of an increased risk of blood clots. Women with a history of pelvic infections should not use IUDs; reinfection is a risk.

**Why use a contraceptive?**
*The bar chart on the left shows the number of deaths (per 100,000 women in the US) caused by childbirth and by use of the combined contraceptive pill. The pill poses the highest risk of serious (and possibly fatal) side effects of all birth control methods. Yet the risk of death from childbirth is always greater, except for women using the pill who are over 35 and smoke. Using a contraceptive prevents the potential health threat of childbirth and the other consequences of unwanted pregnancy.*

# BARRIER METHODS OF CONTRACEPTION

Barrier methods of contraception prevent pregnancy by blocking or killing sperm so that they cannot reach the egg to fertilize it. Barrier methods include the male condom, the female condom, the diaphragm, the cervical cap, and the vaginal sponge, all used with spermicides. The most common cause of pregnancy among women relying on barrier methods is a failure to use them.

### The male condom
*The male condom is a method of birth control that is particularly useful for spontaneous intercourse and for preventing the spread of sexually transmitted disease. Worldwide, an estimated 40 million couples regularly use condoms. A condom is a thin latex rubber tube with one closed end designed to cover the erect penis during sex and to contain ejaculated semen, preventing it from reaching the egg. Condoms are made in different thicknesses and colors and some have special textures or types of tips. Some condoms are prelubricated and some are treated with a spermicide.*

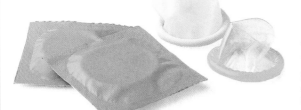

### The female condom
*Work is under way in the US to produce an acceptable female condom. Like the male condom, one type of female condom (below) is made of a thin rubber tube, but it has a ring at either end. One of these rings is closed and is inserted into the vagina so that it covers the cervix, much like a diaphragm. The other end is open and fits around the opening of the vagina and vulva. The female condom provides women with extra protection against sexually transmitted diseases.*

### Spermicides
*Spermicides are substances that chemically destroy sperm. Used alone, they are not very reliable. They are usually used to increase the effectiveness of other contraceptives such as condoms, diaphragms, and caps. However, spermicides may offer some additional protection against sexually transmitted diseases and cancer of the cervix. This seems to be particularly true of nonoxynol 9, an ingredient in most spermicides. Spermicides are available as creams, gels, foams, or suppositories.*

### The vaginal sponge
*The vaginal sponge (below) is made of absorbent polyurethane foam impregnated with the spermicide nonoxynol 9. You must moisten the sponge to activate the spermicide, then push it high into your vagina. It must be left in place for at least 6 hours after intercourse. The advantages of the sponge are that it can be purchased over-the-counter, it is simple to use, and it can be inserted at any time from a few seconds to 24 hours before intercourse. Its main action is not as a barrier but as a carrier of spermicide, and it can easily be displaced. Its failure rate is relatively high.*

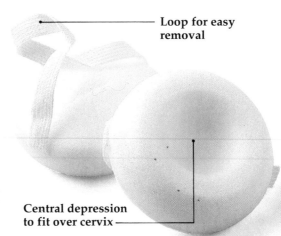

Loop for easy removal

Central depression to fit over cervix

### WARNING
To be used effectively, a condom must be put on before genital-to-genital contact, because sperm can leak out of an erect penis before ejaculation. A condom may leak or rupture if there is no space at the sealed end to contain the semen, or if it is damaged while it is being put on. Leakage may also occur if the man does not withdraw his penis before it becomes flaccid. Another hazard is that oil-based products such as petroleum jelly and baby oil can break down rubber very quickly. If you use a vaginal lubricant, buy one specially developed for use with condoms.

## THE DIAPHRAGM AND THE CERVICAL CAP

Although the diaphragm is often called a cap, the two terms refer to different types of vaginal barrier contraceptives. The diaphragm is the most popular version because most women find it easier to insert. However, caps have some advantages over the diaphragm in certain instances. Women with poor vaginal muscle tone can use them, the male partner does not feel them, they do not reduce vaginal sensation, and they are unlikely to trigger bladder problems. However, to use a cap you must have a certain type of cervix– not too big or too small, for example – and be able to feel your cervix so that you can insert the cap properly. It is necessary to use a spermicide with both diaphragms and caps to be as safe as possible. One disadvantage of both diaphragms and caps is that they must be fitted by a doctor. However, the fitting is an opportunity for you to learn how to insert them correctly. As with other barrier methods, diaphragms and caps and the spermicides used with them offer some protection against some sexually transmitted diseases.

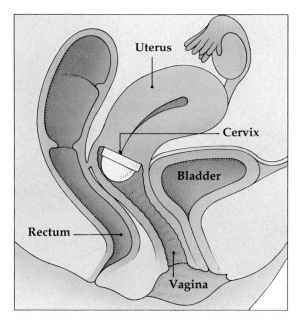

### The cervical cap
*The cervical cap is shaped like a thimble and is designed to fit tightly over the cervix. Cervical caps adhere to the cervix by suction and may therefore provide a better barrier against sperm than the diaphragm. They should always be used with a spermicide.*

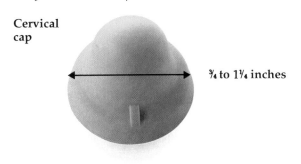

**Cervical cap**

**¾ to 1¼ inches**

### The diaphragm
*Diaphragms are designed to lie diagonally across the cervix and much of the front wall of the vagina. In theory, the muscles of the vagina hold the diaphragm in place, preventing sperm from passing into the cervix. However, the vagina tends to "balloon" during intercourse, sometimes permitting a pool of sperm to remain in the vagina. This is in part why use of a spermicide is necessary with a diaphragm. Use of a spermicide also provides further protection against some sexually transmitted diseases.*

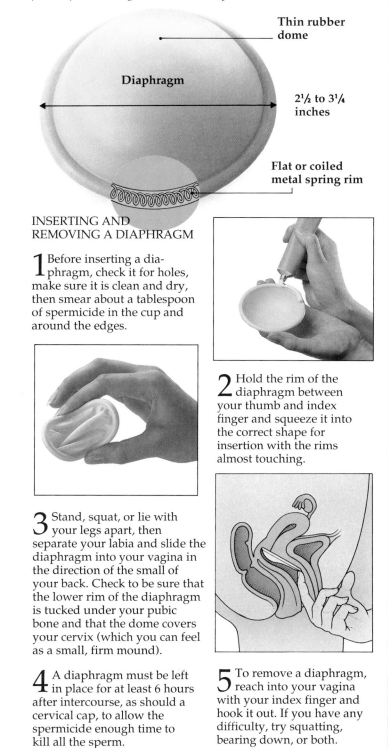

**Thin rubber dome**

**Diaphragm**

**2½ to 3¼ inches**

**Flat or coiled metal spring rim**

### INSERTING AND REMOVING A DIAPHRAGM

1 Before inserting a diaphragm, check it for holes, make sure it is clean and dry, then smear about a tablespoon of spermicide in the cup and around the edges.

2 Hold the rim of the diaphragm between your thumb and index finger and squeeze it into the correct shape for insertion with the rims almost touching.

3 Stand, squat, or lie with your legs apart, then separate your labia and slide the diaphragm into your vagina in the direction of the small of your back. Check to be sure that the lower rim of the diaphragm is tucked under your pubic bone and that the dome covers your cervix (which you can feel as a small, firm mound).

4 A diaphragm must be left in place for at least 6 hours after intercourse, as should a cervical cap, to allow the spermicide enough time to kill all the sperm.

5 To remove a diaphragm, reach into your vagina with your index finger and hook it out. If you have any difficulty, try squatting, bearing down, or both.

# HORMONAL CONTRACEPTION

Hormonal contraception – taking hormones to prevent pregnancy – began 30 years ago when the combined contraceptive pill was approved in the US.

## The combined contraceptive pill

The combined contraceptive pill contains synthetic forms of the two female sex hormones estrogen and progesterone. It works by preventing ovulation, an action backed up by other means. The hormones also cause a thickening of cervical secretions and a reduction in the ability of the uterine lining to receive a fertilized egg (as well as interference with the action of the fallopian tubes, inhibiting transport of sperm and eggs).

Women who use the combined pill derive several benefits. Used properly, it is the most effective form of birth control available, it is convenient, and it does not interfere in any way with sexual intercourse. It can also reduce menstrual problems such as heavy bleeding, anemia, menstrual pain (dysmenorrhea), irregular periods, and pain during ovulation. The combined pill can also have a protective effect against more serious health problems, including certain types of pelvic inflammatory disease, ovarian cysts, and ovarian and uterine cancer.

However, in some women, the combined pill can cause troublesome side effects that may mimic symptoms of pregnancy – including missed periods, between-period spotting (bleeding), headache, weight gain, loss of sexual desire, nausea, depression, leg cramps, skin problems, and breast tenderness.

The combined pill also carries a small risk of more serious health problems, such as liver and gallbladder diseases and strokes and heart attacks. The risk of cardiovascular problems is greater with age and obesity; if you smoke cigarettes; or if you have diabetes, high cholesterol levels, or high blood pressure.

### WARNING

The combined pill is effective if you take it within 12 hours of your usual time, that is, within 36 hours of your last pill. If you miss one, take it as soon as you remember and take the next one on time. If you miss taking the pill for more than 12 hours, use an additional contraceptive method for 14 days. Take extra contraceptive precautions if you vomit within 3 hours or have severe diarrhea within 12 hours of taking the pill because it may not have been absorbed properly. Use a backup method or talk to your doctor if you are taking antibiotics; they can increase the failure rate.

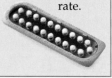

## THE COMBINED PILL AND CANCER

Most doctors agree that the pill prevents more cancers than it causes. Cancers of the ovaries and endometrium (the lining of the uterus) occur less frequently in women who take the combined pill. However, some studies suggest a possible increase in the incidence of cervical cancer, particularly in women who have been taking the pill for more than 5 years. There may also be a small additional risk of breast cancer in some women taking the combined pill, which is more likely in those taking it for a long time. It is important to understand that these findings are inconsistent and most studies have found no increased risk of breast or cervical cancer.

**Breast cancer**
*The largest study done showed no greater risk of breast cancer in women who used the pill. Nor was there an increased risk among women using the pill who had other high-risk factors – for example, a family history of breast cancer.*

**Liver cancer**
*Limited, unconfirmed evidence suggests that taking the pill may slightly increase the risk of liver cancer.*

**Cervical cancer**
*A review of studies since 1980 suggests that the risk of dysplasia, a condition that can develop into cervical cancer, may double after a woman takes the pill for 8 to 10 years. However, other studies cast doubt on the role of the pill in increasing the risk of cervical cancer.*

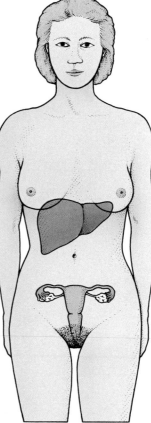

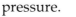

**Ovarian cancer**
*The risk of ovarian cancer is halved after taking the pill for 4 years; this protection lasts for 15 years.*

**Endometrial cancer**
*The risk of endometrial (uterine) cancer is reduced by up to 60 percent after taking the pill for 4 to 5 years. This protection lasts for 15 years.*

## The minipill

The minipill, known as the progestin-only contraceptive pill (because it doesn't contain an estrogenlike drug), has fewer side effects than the combined pill. However, doctors are still unclear about exactly how the minipill works. While the combined pill totally suppresses ovulation, the minipill does not always do so, with the result that menstruation can be less predictable and erratic bleeding may occur. The minipill is thought to prevent conception by thickening cervical secretions, altering the uterine lining, and interfering with conditions in the fallopian tubes – similar to the backup actions of the combined pill. The minipill is usually recommended for women who should not take the combined pill, including smokers older than 35, women who are breast-feeding, diabetics, and women with high blood pressure.

If you are taking the minipill, it is important to remember that you must take it at the same time each day. It can cease to be effective if you take it as little as 3 hours later than your regular time. If you forget to take your minipill, take it as soon as you remember and use extra precautions for 48 hours. If you miss two or more minipills in a row, immediately start using your backup method. Start taking your minipill again right away and take two a day for 2 days.

## NEW AND FUTURE HORMONAL CONTRACEPTIVE METHODS

Several new ways of delivering female hormones are being developed in an effort to increase their contraceptive effectiveness, reduce their side effects, and make them easier to use.

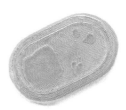

**Hormonally impregnated IUD**
*There is one intrauterine device (IUD) available that contains a synthetic progesterone. Its duration of action is 1 year. During this time, the hormone is slowly released into the uterus.*

**The vaginal ring**
*The vaginal ring, which is still being tested in the US, is made of silicon-based rubber with a hollow inner core. This core is filled with a progesteronelike hormone. The ring is inserted into the vagina, where it delivers the hormone continuously. It can be left in place for as long as 3 months. Because it is soft and compressible, it does not interfere with sexual intercourse.*

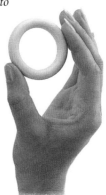

**Skin patches**
*Adhesive patches impregnated with estrogenlike and progesteronelike hormones are currently being developed as a form of contraception. They can be used to deliver the hormones continuously over a few days or weeks. As the hormones are released, they pass through the skin to be absorbed by the bloodstream.*

**Morning-after pill**
*The morning-after pill contains very high doses of estrogen and progesterone and is used to prevent pregnancy shortly after unprotected intercourse has taken place. It works by stopping a fertilized egg from implanting in the uterus, but it must be taken within 72 hours of intercourse. It is under study and currently is not available in the US. However, certain hormones currently available for other uses may also be used as morning-after contraceptives.*

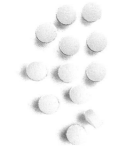

**Hormonal injections**
*Injectable contraceptives contain a progesteronelike hormone in liquid suspension that controls release of the hormone. They are injected deep into a buttock muscle and last for 1 to 6 months. Testing of this technology has already begun, but injections are not currently approved in the US.*

**Hormonal implants**
*The implants that have recently become available in the US contain progestin – the same synthetic hormone used in some birth control pills – in slow-release capsules. Six implants, which are almost the size of matches, are inserted under the skin on the inside of the upper part of your arm. They deliver a constant supply of the hormone for a period of up to 5 years, with 99.3 percent effectiveness. The implant is a convenient contraceptive alternative, but may cause spotting.*

# ASK YOUR DOCTOR
## CONTRACEPTION

**Q** **I am going to stop taking the pill and get a diaphragm instead. Will douching work until I can get a diaphragm fitted?**

**A** No. Douching, or washing out the vagina after intercourse, is not an effective contraceptive method. Sperm move quickly into the cervix, uterus, and fallopian tubes, and douching does not reach any of these areas. Douching can also leave you more vulnerable to vaginal and pelvic infections.

**Q** **I forgot to take my diaphragm with me on a trip last weekend. My husband used the withdrawal method instead. How effective is this method?**

**A** The withdrawal method is unreliable because the timing of withdrawal can be difficult and because sperm can leak from a penis as soon as it becomes erect – not only during orgasm. Couples who use this method often end up with an unwanted pregnancy.

**Q** **I am 23 years old and don't want to have children yet. I can't take the pill because I had a blood clot last year. Am I a good candidate for an IUD?**

**A** An IUD (intrauterine device) is a good method of contraception, but it carries a risk of ectopic pregnancy (development of an embryo outside of the uterus) and pelvic inflammatory disease. Because these conditions can cause infertility, an IUD is not recommended for women who want to have children. Among your options are the diaphragm, cervical cap, or condoms with spermicide. Hormonal contraceptives may not be recommended for you.

# NATURAL FAMILY PLANNING

There are three ways to identify a woman's fertile time – the temperature method, calendar method, and cervical mucus method. These methods can be used to determine when to have intercourse if you wish to conceive or when to avoid intercourse to prevent conception. To use any of these methods properly, you must have training from your doctor or family planning clinic. None of these methods has proved to be consistently reliable as a means of contraception. None of these methods is reliable for women who have irregular cycles.

## The temperature method

Women using the temperature method monitor their temperature every day and record it on a chart. For most women, temperature taken with an oral thermometer ranges from 96 to 98 °F (35.6 to 36.7 °C) before ovulation. It then increases to between 97 and 99 °F (36.1 to 37.2 °C) immediately after ovulation, and stays at a slightly higher level until just before their next period.

If you are trying to avoid conception, you should wait 3 days after the rise in temperature to have intercourse. The temperature method accurately indicates when ovulation has occurred, but it does not help you predict when it is about to occur. You must wait until the second half of each cycle (after ovulation) to have intercourse.

**Choosing a thermometer**
*Because the changes in temperature are small, it is best to use a large-scale, easy-to-read thermometer that only registers from 96 to 100 °F (35.6 to 37.8 °C).*

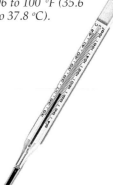

**Taking your temperature**
*To use the temperature method correctly, you should take your temperature at the same time each day. The best time is the moment you wake up in the morning, before you get out of bed, talk, eat, drink, or smoke. In addition, you should keep the thermometer in your mouth for a full 5 minutes.*

## The calendar method

To use the calendar method effectively, you must record the number of days that pass from the first day of one period to the first day of the next period for a full year (the day bleeding starts is recorded as day 1). Ovulation reliably occurs 12 to 15 days before the onset of your period. Doctors suggest that women with very reliable 28-day cycles will have fertile days between days 9 and 18 and women with 25- to 35-day cycles will have fertile days from day 7 to day 21. Women with irregular cycles who do not wish to conceive will have very few "safe" days. Failures are common when the cycle changes, such as during the late 30s and early 40s, after childbirth, during times of stress, or with weight fluctuations. The calendar method is the least precise of the three natural planning methods.

## The cervical mucus method

Ovulation can be predicted by carefully examining your vaginal secretions every day to detect changes in the quantity, appearance, and quality of your cervical mucus. Immediately before and for about 3 days after ovulation, mucus becomes more profuse, clear, and slippery. The cervical mucus method (also known as the Billings method) is the most accurate of the three natural family planning methods. Each day you need to chart whether your vagina feels dry or wet, whether the secretions look clear or cloudy, and whether the texture is sticky and pasty, or slippery. You can feel the secretions between your finger and thumb. Intercourse must be avoided from the earliest time of fertile (slippery and clear) mucus until *after* it has become more thick and pasty.

**HOW LONG DO SPERM LIVE?**

Evidence suggests that sperm can survive for up to 7 days in the female reproductive tract and an egg can be fertilized for up to 24 hours after it has been released. A couple who uses natural family planning to prevent conception should therefore avoid intercourse for a period beginning at least 7 days before the estimated day of ovulation and at least 2 days after that day.

### THE THREE-CHECK METHOD

Combining all three methods of natural family planning can give you the most reliable indication of your fertile period. The charts below illustrate the types of readings to expect from all three methods used alone and combined. The external signs that are recorded reflect the effects that hormonal changes have on your body throughout your menstrual cycle.

**Combining methods** — Ovulation ▼

| 1 | 2 | 3 | 4 | 5 | 6 | 7 | 8 | 9 | 10 | 11 | 12 | 13 | 14 | 15 | 16 | 17 | 18 | 19 | 20 | 21 | 22 | 23 | 24 | 25 | 26 | 27 | 28 |
|---|---|---|---|---|---|---|---|---|----|----|----|----|----|----|----|----|----|----|----|----|----|----|----|----|----|----|----|

Fertile days

**Calendar method**

Menstruation — Fertile days

**Cervical mucus method**

Menstruation | Dry | Cloudy, pasty, thick | Clear, slippery, profuse, wet | Dry, scant, pasty, thick

Fertile days

**Temperature method**

Menstruation — Fertile days

°F: 98.4, 98.2, 98.0, 97.8, 97.6, 97.4, 97.2, 97.0

°C: 36.9, 36.8, 36.7, 36.6, 36.5, 36.4, 36.3, 36.2, 36.1

# INTRAUTERINE DEVICES

Currently only two types of IUDs are available in the US, one that is impregnated with a progesteronelike hormonal drug (see NEW AND FUTURE HORMONAL CONTRACEPTIVE METHODS on page 69) and one that contains copper.

The primary mechanism of action for both IUDs is spermicidal – the inflammatory reaction to the foreign body in the uterus kills the sperm. Secondarily, the devices may prevent implantation of an egg in the uterine wall.

## Benefits and risks

The advantages of IUDs are that they are convenient, are long-lasting, give constant protection, and do not interfere with sexual intercourse in any way. Disadvantages include side effects such as cramps, spotting, and heavier or longer menstrual periods, and the fact that they must be inserted or removed by a doctor. Occasionally, IUDs can also perforate the uterus or cervix, increase the risk of ectopic pregnancy, and cause infection of the uterine lining or fallopian tubes, which may lead to sterility. For this reason, they are not recommended for women who may be planning to have children at a future time.

# CONTRACEPTIVE DRUGS NOW UNDER STUDY

In the foreseeable future we may be able to add a male pill, a contraceptive vaccine, and a drug that induces abortion to the list of birth control methods that are available.

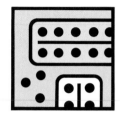

**Male pills**
*Several types of male pills (and other technologies) are under investigation in the US. Preparations currently being studied act by interfering with sperm formation in various ways. The effects of these male pills are being investigated. The pills are highly experimental and unavailable to the public.*

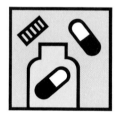

**Contraceptive vaccines**
*Three types of contraceptive vaccines are currently being evaluated. They probably will be effective only in women. One of the vaccines activates the woman's immune system against sperm and another activates it against eggs. The third vaccine activates the woman's immune system against the hormone that prevents menstruation in women when they have just become pregnant. This prevents the fertilized egg from implanting into the lining of the uterus. A major problem with this form of contraception is its irreversibility.*

**RU-486**
*Early studies with RU-486 (mifepristone) have shown that it can induce abortion in women who are up to 6 weeks pregnant if it is given in conjunction with prostaglandins – drugs that cause uterine contractions. The female hormone progesterone is needed to maintain pregnancy. RU-486, which resembles the hormone, works by blocking the effect of progesterone in the uterus. Prolonged bleeding and cramping seem to be the main side effects of the drug. RU-486 is currently available only in France, West Germany, and China.*

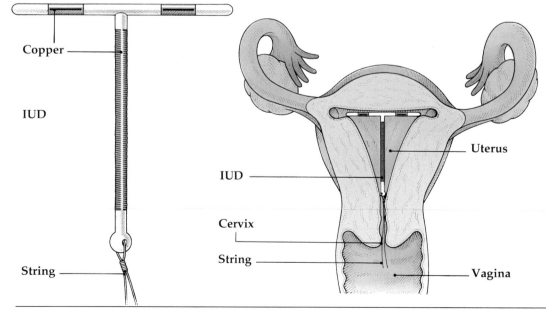

Copper

IUD

String

IUD

Cervix

String

Uterus

IUD

Vagina

**Using an IUD**
*All IUDs have a string attached to them that runs through your cervix and into your vagina. You can make sure the device is in place by feeling for the string with your finger – something you should do after each period because an IUD can come out. The string also enables your doctor to remove the device once its effectiveness is complete – after 1 year for currently used progesterone-containing IUDs and 3 to 5 years for copper-containing IUDs.*

# CASE HISTORY
# A COMPLETE FAMILY

R EBECCA AND JOHN **have used a variety of contraceptive methods during their marriage. They have carefully planned the births of their three children and have agreed that they do not want a larger family. Rebecca is reluctant to use contraceptives for her remaining 10 or more fertile years. They decided to ask their doctor for advice.**

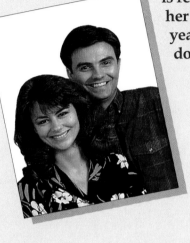

## PERSONAL DETAILS
**Names** Rebecca and John Newman
**Ages** 38 and 36, respectively
**Occupations** John is an engineer in an automotive plant and Rebecca is a full-time homemaker.
**Family** They have three children ages 15, 8, and 2.

## MEDICAL BACKGROUND
Both Rebecca and John have always been healthy. For many years Rebecca took the combined contraceptive pill between pregnancies. Three years ago, she decided to use a barrier method and chose the diaphragm with spermicide.

## THE CONSULTATION
Rebecca and John go together to see the doctor. Once he is sure that they do not want to have more children, the doctor explains to them the possible alternatives for controlling their fertility. Rebecca says that she is tired of using the diaphragm, so he outlines the options open to them involving sterilization.

## THE OPTIONS
The doctor explains that the two possible alternatives are male sterilization (vasectomy) or female sterilization (tubal ligation). He says that, for John, sterilization would be a simple procedure in which each vas deferens (a tube that carries sperm from a testicle to the penis during ejaculation) would be cut and tied. This procedure would require a local anesthetic and one small incision into John's scrotum. In contrast, the doctor explains that, for Rebecca, the sterilization procedure would require making an incision in her abdomen and then cutting her fallopian tubes while looking through a laparoscope (an instrument used for looking into the abdomen). This procedure is usually performed in an outpatient operating room.

Having explained the procedures, their rates of failure, and the rates of complications, he tells Rebecca and John that the decision is theirs.

## THE OUTCOME
The Newmans decide that John should have a vasectomy because the procedure seems to carry less risk. John has the operation a week later and is back at work the next day. Aside from a black and blue area at the site of the incision in his scrotum and some mild discomfort for a few days, John is fine. Rebecca continues to use her diaphragm for 3 more months until John's sperm count has registered zero on three consecutive occasions. They find that, in the following years, their sexual relationship is enhanced because the possibility of pregnancy is gone and they do not have to worry about contraception.

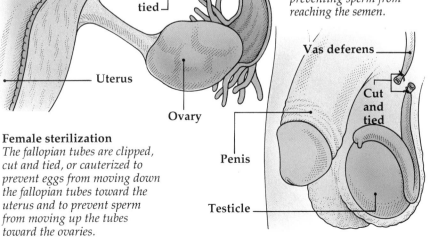

**Female sterilization**
*The fallopian tubes are clipped, cut and tied, or cauterized to prevent eggs from moving down the fallopian tubes toward the uterus and to prevent sperm from moving up the tubes toward the ovaries.*

**Male sterilization**
*Each vas deferens, which carries sperm from a testicle to the penis, is clipped, cut and tied, or cauterized, thereby preventing sperm from reaching the semen.*

# CHAPTER FOUR

# HEALTH PROBLEMS AND DISORDERS

## INTRODUCTION

WOMEN'S SYMPTOMS

INFERTILITY

PROBLEMS OF ADOLESCENCE

URINARY TRACT PROBLEMS

MENSTRUAL PROBLEMS

BREAST DISORDERS

SEXUALLY TRANSMITTED DISEASES

MENOPAUSAL PROBLEMS

UTERINE, OVARIAN, AND VAGINAL DISORDERS

PROBLEMS OF THE OLDER WOMAN

ANXIETY AND DEPRESSION

D O YOU SOMETIMES feel that you just don't have time to pay attention to every physical symptom you notice, as long as it doesn't interfere with your activities? It is important to remember that your body may be telling you something. Just as fixing a minor problem in your home or car can prevent a major repair from being necessary in the future, treatment of today's minor symptoms may benefit your health over the long term. Some general symptoms are nothing to worry about or you can treat them yourself. However, all women should be able to recognize the warning signs that could indicate a serious disorder. In this chapter we outline the symptoms and signs of many conditions that usually or always affect only women. These disorders represent a large part of the health problems for which women go to their doctors. Among the typical problems are such conditions as cystitis, pelvic inflammatory disease (which affects more than 1 million American women each year), menopausal problems, and cancers of the breast, ovary, uterus, and cervix (which together account for more than 40 percent of all cancers in women). Some of the problems women have in common with men – such as anxiety, depression, and cardiovascular disease – are also discussed.

Describing your symptoms accurately to your doctor is a great help to him or her in diagnosing your problem. An experienced doctor can often reach a diagnosis simply by listening to you describe your symptoms. He or she may recommend further tests. A laparoscopic examination, for example, enables your doctor to see the organs in your abdominal cavity. Mammography provides an X-ray of your breast tissue. With the results of such tests, your doctor can investigate the cause of your symptoms, determine how a disorder may progress, and talk to you about ways to treat it.

This chapter opens with a section on women's symptoms that discusses problems many women are likely to encounter. Much of the chapter focuses on specific parts of a woman's body, such as the breasts, genitourinary tract, and reproductive system, and the special problems that may affect them. There are also sections on the causes and effects of sexually transmitted diseases, as well as guidance concerning problems of adolescence and problems of the older woman. You can learn about the treatments that are available for many conditions and the ways in which you can reduce your risk of some disorders. The chapter also includes information about the problems of infertility.

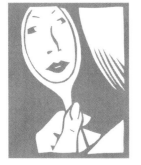

# WOMEN'S SYMPTOMS

A TENDER BREAST, an itch, a bump, or a discharge – is it a minor symptom that will disappear overnight or is it the first indication of a serious illness? In the course of a hectic life, you still need to take the time to seek medical advice for any symptom that persists without an apparent cause.

A woman's body undergoes significant changes during the years from puberty through menopause (see THE FERTILE YEARS on page 16). Each stage is accompanied by psychological adjustments to the changes and some symptoms. Every woman benefits from knowing what these changes are, how and why they occur, and how to distinguish normal from abnormal symptoms.

**Taking care of yourself**
*Many women believe they are too busy to pay attention to each and every symptom they have. Instead, they dismiss them as minor or unavoidable. It is true that some symptoms are caused by hormonal changes during the*

*menstrual cycle, pregnancy, or menopause. However, any symptom that makes you uncomfortable should prompt you to see your doctor. Never ignore any new or worsening symptom.*

## NORMAL SYMPTOMS

During her fertile years, a woman experiences regular monthly changes brought about by her menstrual cycle. Not only do women shed their uterine lining at the beginning of each cycle, but they experience hormonal peaks and valleys that can affect their body weight (because of fluctuations in water balance),

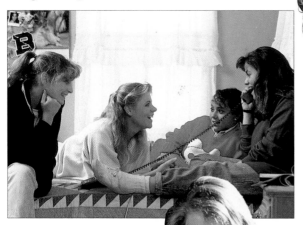

the appearance of skin and hair, and their emotional state. These hormonal changes are modified, as are the symptoms they produce, when you use a contraceptive that contains hormones.

Around 80 percent of women become pregnant at least once in their lives. The hormonal adjustments that accompany pregnancy, childbirth, and breast-feeding cause changes in the body, as do the direct physical stresses of childbearing. Menopause also brings hormonal changes, the signs and symptoms of which may be difficult to distinguish from those caused by the psychological stresses of daily life. Finally, aging itself causes gradual changes in your body.

## Staying aware

As you move from one stage of your life to another, observe what is happening to your body and discuss the changes with your doctor. He or she can let you know whether the changes are to be expected or may be signs of trouble. Women who are educated about the normal changes their bodies undergo, such as irregular periods in the years before menopause, are better equipped to cope with the changes as healthy occurrences.

## Breast symptoms

When the breasts begin to develop in adolescence, they form swellings of about 1 inch in diameter beneath the skin. The breasts may develop amazingly quickly, or more gradually. They will probably be sore at times. In adolescent girls it is also quite common, and normal, for the breasts to be slightly different in size. The size and shape of the breasts of a mature woman also vary to some degree at different times in her life.

Many women find that their breasts become enlarged and tender just before each menstrual period, and sometimes they can feel firm nodules within their breasts. If nodules appear and then disappear after your menstrual period, which is usually the case, they are no cause for concern. Tender breasts and nipples can also be one of the first signs of pregnancy, and a milky discharge from a nipple may occur in late pregnancy. If you notice discharge or a lump at other times, discuss it with your doctor.

**Talking to your doctor**
*It is ideal to have a doctor (such as a family doctor or internist) for general health care as well as a gynecologist for care and treatment of your reproductive system. Don't be embarrassed to discuss any problem or concern. Speaking frankly with your doctor is essential to your health.*

**THE MENOPAUSE**

As you approach your 50th birthday, you should anticipate the onset of the menopause. In fact, 52 is the average age of onset, but you may notice symptoms such as irregular periods in your late 30s or early 40s and your periods may stop anytime from the mid 40s to the mid 50s. You may also have other menopausal symptoms such as hot flashes, vaginal dryness, skin changes, and anxiety (see HOW DO I RECOGNIZE THE MENOPAUSE? on page 32).

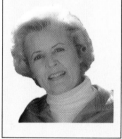

# WHEN SHOULD I CONSULT MY DOCTOR?

Serious illnesses often start with seemingly minor symptoms. Most serious illnesses are more easily treated when they are detected early. If you have any of the problems discussed here, talk to your doctor without delay.

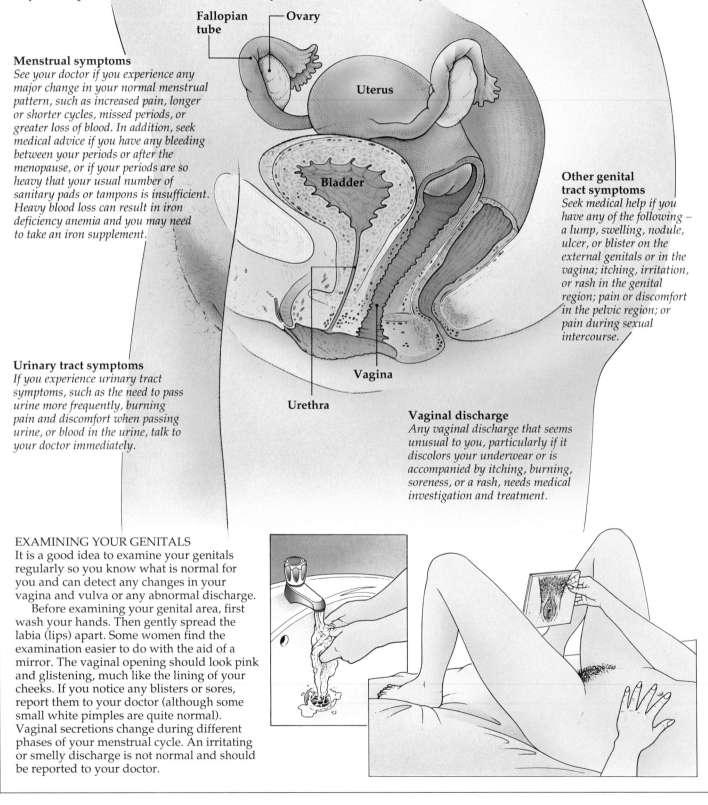

**Menstrual symptoms**

*See your doctor if you experience any major change in your normal menstrual pattern, such as increased pain, longer or shorter cycles, missed periods, or greater loss of blood. In addition, seek medical advice if you have any bleeding between your periods or after the menopause, or if your periods are so heavy that your usual number of sanitary pads or tampons is insufficient. Heavy blood loss can result in iron deficiency anemia and you may need to take an iron supplement.*

**Fallopian tube** — **Ovary**

**Uterus**

**Bladder**

**Other genital tract symptoms**

*Seek medical help if you have any of the following – a lump, swelling, nodule, ulcer, or blister on the external genitals or in the vagina; itching, irritation, or rash in the genital region; pain or discomfort in the pelvic region; or pain during sexual intercourse.*

**Vagina**

**Urethra**

**Urinary tract symptoms**

*If you experience urinary tract symptoms, such as the need to pass urine more frequently, burning pain and discomfort when passing urine, or blood in the urine, talk to your doctor immediately.*

**Vaginal discharge**

*Any vaginal discharge that seems unusual to you, particularly if it discolors your underwear or is accompanied by itching, burning, soreness, or a rash, needs medical investigation and treatment.*

EXAMINING YOUR GENITALS

It is a good idea to examine your genitals regularly so you know what is normal for you and can detect any changes in your vagina and vulva or any abnormal discharge.

Before examining your genital area, first wash your hands. Then gently spread the labia (lips) apart. Some women find the examination easier to do with the aid of a mirror. The vaginal opening should look pink and glistening, much like the lining of your cheeks. If you notice any blisters or sores, report them to your doctor (although some small white pimples are quite normal). Vaginal secretions change during different phases of your menstrual cycle. An irritating or smelly discharge is not normal and should be reported to your doctor.

### Changes in breast appearance
*If there are any changes in the size, shape, or color of your breasts, see your doctor immediately. Puckering of the skin or an "orange peel" appearance may indicate a tumor under the skin. Redness or swelling of any part of the breast may indicate an underlying abscess or infection.*

### Changes in nipple appearance
*See your doctor promptly about any change in the size, shape, or color of a nipple. Such a change may indicate a tumor beneath the nipple or a disease of the nipple itself. If you notice that your nipple has become inverted when it previously protruded, talk with your doctor.*

### A lump in your breast
*Any lump in your breast, whatever your age, could be an indication of cancer. Four out of five breast lumps are harmless, but only a thorough medical examination can definitely rule out a malignant tumor.*

### Breast pain
*Many women experience breast pain and tenderness just before their periods or during pregnancy because of changes in the glands in the breast. Tell your doctor about any severe or persistent pain.*

### Discharge from a nipple
*Discharge from a nipple is usually the result of increased levels of the hormone prolactin, which stimulates milk production. This increase is normal in late pregnancy. It can also occur after a miscarriage or an abortion. However, discharge may also be a side effect of some drugs, or a sign of breast infection, cysts, or even cancer. Consult your doctor if you have a discharge and are not pregnant.*

## EXAMINING YOUR BREASTS
It is important for every woman to examine her breasts regularly. The best time to do this is at the end of each menstrual period when your breasts are the least tender and cystic (lumpy).

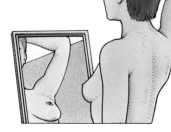

**1** Stand in front of a mirror and look at the size, shape, and color of your breasts and nipples.

**2** Raise your arms above your head and again check for any changes in the size or shape of your breasts and nipples.

**3** Next, lie down and perform a manual breast examination. With your nipple as the center, divide your breasts into imaginary quadrants.

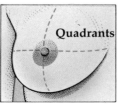

**Quadrants**

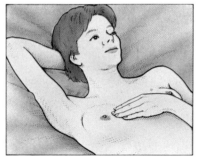

**4** Using the pads of your fingers, make firm circular movements over each quadrant, feeling for any unusual lumps or areas of tenderness. Use your left hand to examine your right breast with your right hand behind your head and vice versa.

**5** When you reach the upper outer quadrant of your breast, continue toward your armpit. Press down in all directions.

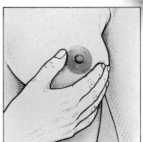

**6** Finally, feel each nipple for any change in size or shape and gently squeeze each to check for any discharge.

# MONITOR YOUR SYMPTOMS
# IRREGULAR VAGINAL BLEEDING

Irregular vaginal bleeding includes irregular menstrual periods and blood loss between normal periods. Sometimes irregular periods are the result of hormonal fluctuations that women experience in adolescence and as the menopause approaches. Bleeding between periods, which may be slight spotting on 1 or 2 days or much heavier bleeding, can be a sign of a serious disorder. Your doctor should investigate the possible cause.

*Is the amount of bleeding the same as that of your normal periods?* NO

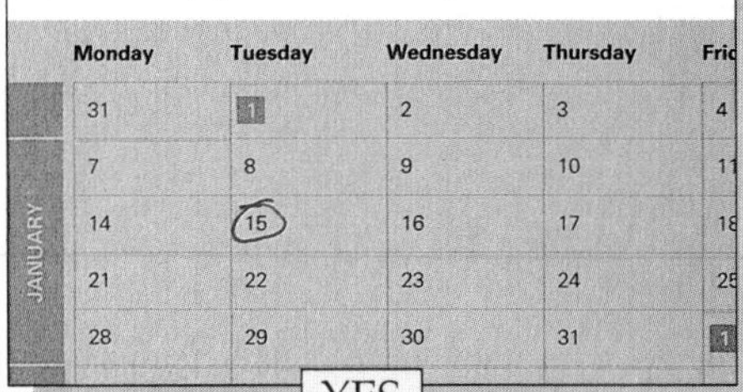

| | Monday | Tuesday | Wednesday | Thursday | Frid |
|---|---|---|---|---|---|
| JANUARY | 31 | 1 | 2 | 3 | 4 |
| | 7 | 8 | 9 | 10 | 11 |
| | 14 | 15 | 16 | 17 | 18 |
| | 21 | 22 | 23 | 24 | 25 |
| | 28 | 29 | 30 | 31 | 1 |

YES

**BEGIN HERE**

**In early pregnancy, spotting is common.**

*Is it possible that you are pregnant?*

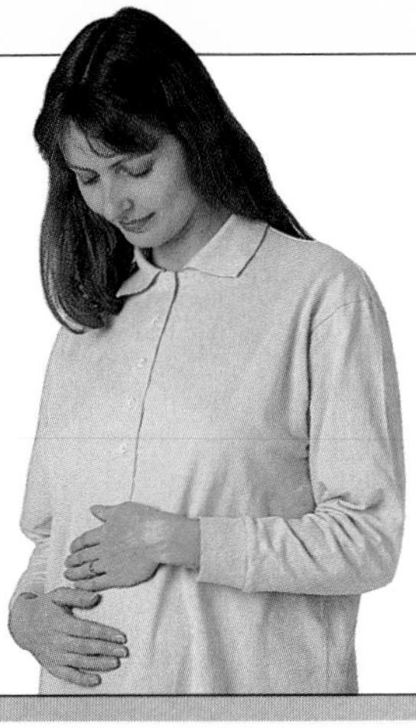

NO

**For the first few years of menstruation, irregular periods are common.**

*Have your periods started just recently?*

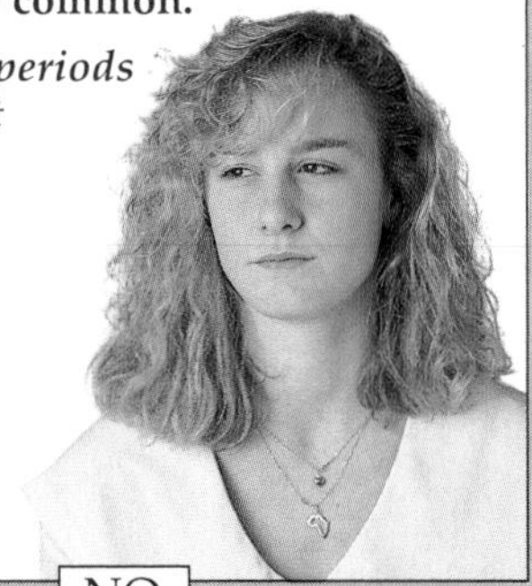

NO

YES

YES

*Action* If you are pregnant, spotting does not indicate a risk to the pregnancy, but you should discuss the spotting with your doctor. Your doctor may advise you to rest until the bleeding stops and may recommend ultrasound scanning to be sure that you do not have an ectopic (tubal) pregnancy or to determine if the embryo is alive.

*Action* Your periods will gradually become regular. However, if you are concerned, see your doctor.

**As you approach menopause, your periods may become irregular.**

*Are you over 40?*

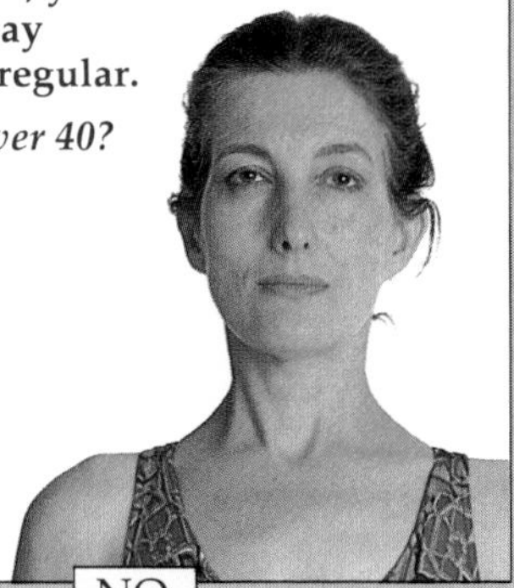

*Action* Although menstrual irregularity is common in premenopausal women, talk to your doctor to ensure that your bleeding falls within a normal pattern for your age.

YES

NO

*Action* Consult your doctor if the period was abnormal in any other way, such as heavier or more painful.

NO

**Having an occasional irregular period is no cause for concern.**

*Have your periods been irregular for more than 2 months?*

YES

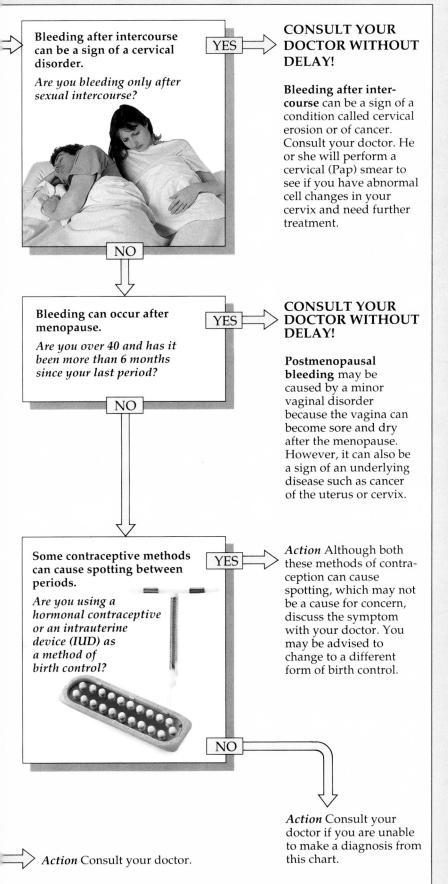

**Bleeding after intercourse can be a sign of a cervical disorder.**

*Are you bleeding only after sexual intercourse?*

YES →

**CONSULT YOUR DOCTOR WITHOUT DELAY!**

**Bleeding after intercourse** can be a sign of a condition called cervical erosion or of cancer. Consult your doctor. He or she will perform a cervical (Pap) smear to see if you have abnormal cell changes in your cervix and need further treatment.

NO ↓

**Bleeding can occur after menopause.**

*Are you over 40 and has it been more than 6 months since your last period?*

YES →

**CONSULT YOUR DOCTOR WITHOUT DELAY!**

**Postmenopausal bleeding** may be caused by a minor vaginal disorder because the vagina can become sore and dry after the menopause. However, it can also be a sign of an underlying disease such as cancer of the uterus or cervix.

NO ↓

**Some contraceptive methods can cause spotting between periods.**

*Are you using a hormonal contraceptive or an intrauterine device (IUD) as a method of birth control?*

YES →

*Action* Although both these methods of contraception can cause spotting, which may not be a cause for concern, discuss the symptom with your doctor. You may be advised to change to a different form of birth control.

NO ↓

*Action* Consult your doctor if you are unable to make a diagnosis from this chart.

→ *Action* Consult your doctor.

## Genital symptoms

Discharge of a white, odorless fluid from your vagina is normal, particularly in adolescence, as long as it does not cause any irritation. The quantity and consistency of this discharge may change according to the phase of your menstrual cycle. At the time of ovulation, your vaginal secretions are thin, almost clear, and copious. During the rest of your cycle, you may have no secretions at all or they may be thick, sticky, and cloudy. If you become pregnant, if you start to take a contraceptive containing the hormone estrogen, or if you have an intrauterine device (IUD) inserted, your vaginal secretions may also change. If a discharge with a foul odor or vaginal itching or burning develops, talk to your doctor about your symptoms.

## Menstrual symptoms

When women discuss the symptoms associated with menstruation, their experiences vary widely. Some women are barely inconvenienced by the menstrual cycle, while others have severe pain and the symptoms of premenstrual syndrome (see PREMENSTRUAL SYNDROME on page 90). Whatever the symptoms, a woman's menstrual pattern is usually consistent from month to month, or nearly so. Most women experience some menstrual disorder at some time in their lives. While irregularities can be symptoms of a serious disease, the vast majority are the result of minor, temporary imbalances in a finely tuned system.

Bleeding lasts an average of 5 days but it may last as little as 2 days or as long as 7 days. The overall cycle may be as short as 21 days or as long as 45 days. Blood loss averages about 1 ounce for each period – four well-soaked tampons or sanitary pads in 24 hours is typical. Learn the characteristics of your normal menstrual pattern, but do not hesitate to talk to your doctor about any distressing physical or emotional symptoms. They may be avoidable. There are several treatment options available for menstrual pain and premenstrual syndrome.

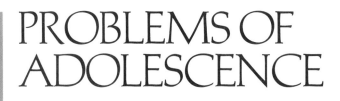

# PROBLEMS OF ADOLESCENCE

O N THE WAY FROM CHILDHOOD to adulthood, an adolescent experiences emotional and physical changes. The onset of puberty causes hormone levels to fluctuate. You may be looking forward to the changes you know will take place in your body. And you may be curious about how your experience compares to that of other young women.

During the years surrounding their first menstrual period, girls are sure to notice changes in their figure, skin, and body hair. As you reach sexual maturity, you will also become more curious about sex. You will spend more time with your friends and explore new social experiences, and you may be exposed to tobacco, alcohol, and other drugs of abuse. Your life is changing quickly, and the more you understand about the changes, the more easily you will adjust.

**You're not alone**
*Talking to friends can be a big help, but if you think your feelings may be more than you can handle, don't be embarrassed to ask an adult you trust for help.*

## THE ONSET OF MENSTRUATION

The onset of menstruation usually causes some minor problems. Your periods may start very early or late, they may be irregular, or you may experience some degree of menstrual pain. In most cases, these problems are not a sign of any disorder; only occasionally do they signal that something is wrong.

**Becoming a woman**
*As you develop from a girl into a woman you will experience many new and often confusing emotions. Sometimes it's difficult to know how your feelings compare with those of others. In a recent poll of US teenagers, almost half said they had trouble coping with stressful situations at home and school. More than 60 percent said they sometimes felt sad and hopeless, and girls were twice as likely as boys to report these feelings.*

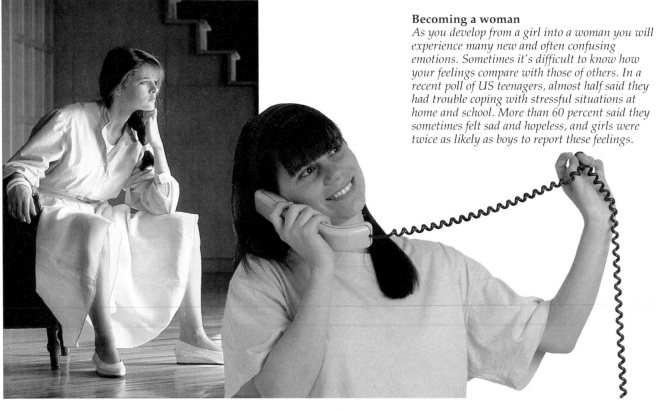

## Delayed menarche

Menarche is the medical term used to describe the onset of menstruation (your first menstrual period). In 95 percent of girls it occurs between 11 and 15. However, it is normal for the start of menstruation to be delayed beyond this age for a variety of reasons. Late onset is often a family characteristic. Girls who are underweight for their age may start menstruating later than the average. Intensive sports activity may also delay the onset of your menstrual periods.

If your periods have not started by the time you are 16, you should talk to your doctor. However, menstruation is the final sign of sexual maturity. If your secondary sexual characteristics (such as your breasts and pubic hair) are developing, it will only be a matter of time before your menstrual periods start too.

## Menstrual pain

Menstrual pain (dysmenorrhea) does not usually occur during the first few periods, but many girls have some discomfort just before and during the first day or two of menstruation once their cycles become more regular. Menstrual pain may result from the body producing excessive amounts of prostaglandins (hormonelike substances), which cause very strong contractions of the muscular wall of the uterus.

The antiprostaglandin painkiller ibuprofen, which you can purchase at a drugstore, is usually effective against mild to moderate pain. In more severe cases, your doctor may prescribe stronger antiprostaglandin painkillers (see TREATING DYSMENORRHEA on page 87). Severe pain may also be triggered by a condition called endometriosis (see page 104).

see TREATING DYSMENORRHEA on page 87; see page 104

### STARTING MENSTRUATION

The menstrual cycle is often irregular during the first 1$\frac{1}{2}$ to 2 years. There may be gaps of 5 or 6 months between periods at first. Keep track of your cycle on a calendar so that you will recognize a regular pattern as it emerges. Even though your periods may be irregular, you can get pregnant. If you are sexually active, talk to a parent, adult friend, or doctor about your sexual activity.

## COPING WITH ACNE

Acne is a skin disorder caused by inflammation of the hair follicles and the sebaceous glands (which open into the hair follicle or directly onto the skin). At puberty, increased hormone levels may make your skin more oily; the oil can block hair follicles and cause pimples. Mild acne can be treated with preparations containing the drug benzoyl peroxide; you can find these products at any drugstore. For more severe cases, your doctor may prescribe an oral antibiotic that you take for several months. Very severe acne may be treated with retinoid drugs. These drugs are used less frequently, however, because they are expensive and can cause side effects such as redness and peeling.

**How does acne occur?**
*A blemish develops when a hair follicle becomes blocked by sebum, an oily substance secreted by the sebaceous gland that opens into the follicle. Bacteria multiply around the plugged follicle, causing it to become red, inflamed, and sometimes filled with pus.*

**Cleaning your skin**
*Washing twice daily with soap and water can remove excess surface oil and help to prevent acne from spreading.*

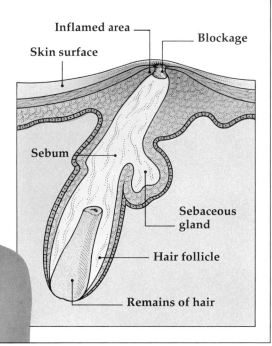

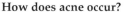

# EATING DISORDERS

Nearly all young girls become more conscious of their weight during adolescence. In the US, as many as one girl in 100 develops such an overwhelming fear of becoming fat that she diets herself down to a weight less than the minimal normal weight for her age and height, a condition known as anorexia nervosa. A different eating disorder called bulimia, characterized by binges of overeating followed by self-induced vomiting or drastic purging with laxatives, also can develop in some girls who are overly concerned about their weight.

## Anorexia nervosa

Doctors have several theories about the possible cause or causes of anorexia nervosa. A high proportion of victims come from close, dominating families and some doctors believe that anorectics may have an unrealistic fear of failure. Other specialists believe that some girls have difficulty coming to terms with the body changes of puberty and they become anorectic to try to keep their childhood figures.

## Bulimia

Bulimics often do their binge eating in secret, going to great lengths to hide their eating habits. After eating huge quantities of food, bulimics usually induce vomiting to relieve the pain of being bloated and to avoid gaining weight. They often become severely depressed after a binge-and-purge episode.

## Treatment of eating disorders

Treatment of an eating disorder usually involves admission to an eating disorder treatment center so that diet can be supervised. The person also undergoes psychotherapy to help resolve emotional problems. Sometimes members of the patient's family take part in therapy sessions to help them understand their roles in the patient's problems.

About half of all anorectics recover within 2 to 3 years, but relapses are common. Up to 10 percent of anorectics eventually die of malnutrition or commit suicide. Bulimia victims often recover, but many relapse weeks or even months after their treatment has ended. They are also at high risk of committing suicide.

**Cultural and social factors**
*Eating disorders occur almost entirely in countries where food is abundant but a slender figure is the ideal. Some experts say that society's fixation with slimness causes some women to diet so extremely that they have tremendous food cravings that can lead to bingeing.*

**Symptoms of anorexia nervosa and bulimia**
*The most obvious manifestation of anorexia is emaciation. As weight loss increases, the young woman becomes tired, weak, and depressed; her skin becomes dry; fine downy hair may grow on her body; and she may lose some hair from her head. In many cases, menstruation stops. If anorexia begins before puberty, the onset of menstruation may be delayed. Girls who have bulimia do not necessarily become very thin, but repeated vomiting can lead to dehydration, weakness, cramps, and damage to the teeth caused by the stomach acid in vomit.*

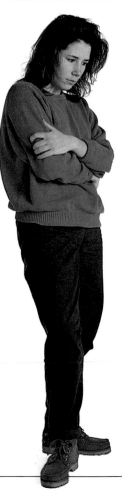

## SOCIAL PRESSURES

As a young woman enters adulthood she is likely to encounter new challenges in her social life, some of which carry potential risks to her health.

## Smoking

It is now well known that smoking can cause lung cancer, heart disease, and other life-threatening disorders, yet many young people start to smoke out of curiosity or because their parents or friends smoke. Smoking is highly addictive. Once you have started it is difficult to stop. A young person may also overlook the unattractive side effects of smoking, such as the smoky odor that stays on the breath and in clothing and the premature wrinkling of a smoker's skin. In addition, a female smoker who becomes pregnant increases the risks that her baby will be born prematurely or with birth defects.

**Just don't start**
*People who have never smoked by the time they are 20 are unlikely to start, but 85 percent of teenagers who smoke become addicted.*

## Alcohol

Alcohol is easily available in our society, but it is a powerful drug that can be both addictive and harmful to your health. Alcohol is a depressant, reducing anxiety and inhibitions. However, the feeling that you are more mentally or physically capable is an illusion. Never drink and drive because even one drink can impair your reaction time and judgment.

## Sexual activity

Once you become sexually active, you accept the responsibility of protecting yourself against unwanted pregnancy and sexually transmitted diseases. Some forms of contraception, such as condoms, provide protection against both possibilities. Young women who are the victims of date rape or other forms of sexual abuse should seek medical attention immediately. Antibiotics will be prescribed to treat possible sexually transmitted diseases and "morning-after" contraception may be required.

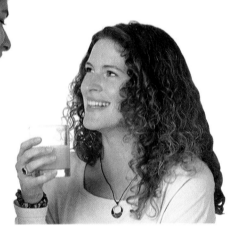

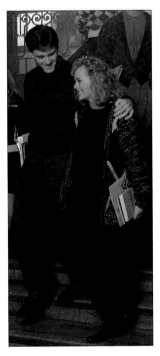

**Social drinking**
*So-called friends may pressure you to drink. You may want to talk to a trusted adult friend or relative about how to say no. More importantly, seek out friends who don't make alcohol the center of their social activities. Doctors tell adults to keep their alcohol intake low.*

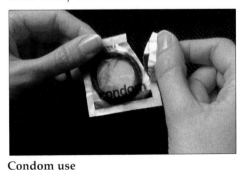

**Condom use**
*If you are sexually active, it is a good idea to carry a condom with you at all times. If you do not have one, insist that your partner get one. Even if you use oral contraceptives, you must use a condom for protection against sexually transmitted disease.*

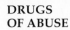

**DRUGS OF ABUSE**

Young people are often exposed to drugs of abuse – many of them illegal. Most of the drugs are highly addictive. Even short-term use can have serious consequences on your physical health and mental well-being. The safest course is always to refuse any drug that is offered to you.

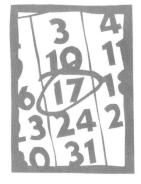

# MENSTRUAL PROBLEMS

**A**LTHOUGH MANY WOMEN have years of relatively trouble-free menstruation, many others encounter a variety of problems with their cycles. These problems include absence of periods (amenorrhea), painful periods (dysmenorrhea), irregular periods, and excessively heavy periods (menorrhagia). Also, many women experience the debilitating premenstrual syndrome as a regular part of their monthly cycles.

Women who have problems with their menstrual cycles should make every effort to find effective relief of their symptoms. It may require overcoming an outdated attitude on the part of some doctors – and some women – that menstrual problems are unavoidable or psychological in origin. In fact, proper medical treatment can often relieve the symptoms of menstrual disorders.

**Causes of amenorrhea**
*Although pregnancy is a common reason for cessation of periods, your periods can stop for a variety of reasons. If you are anxious or depressed, your hormonal balance may be disrupted, which can lead to amenorrhea. Women who exercise frequently and strenuously may stop menstruating. In older women, periods stop with the menopause.*

## AMENORRHEA

There are two types of amenorrhea – primary amenorrhea, which means that menstrual periods have never occurred at all, and secondary amenorrhea, which means periods have not occurred for 3 months or more. Primary amenorrhea is difficult to define in a young woman because the age of onset of menstruation is so variable. Primary amenorrhea is often a family characteristic. It can also be caused by being underweight. However, there are several rare genetic, hormonal, or physical causes that should be investigated if a girl has not started menstruating at 16 years of age.

### Secondary amenorrhea

If a sexually active woman stops menstruating, pregnancy is the most likely cause. It must be considered first, especially if the woman is taking any drugs, because some drugs can be dangerous to the developing fetus and their use must be discontinued. Other possible causes of secondary amenorrhea include lactation, menopause, stress, some nervous system disorders, anorexia nervosa, hormonal disorders, and some drugs. If your menstrual periods stop, consult your doctor. If there is often a gap of a few months between your periods, see the symptom chart IRREGULAR VAGINAL BLEEDING on page 80.

## TREATING DYSMENORRHEA

Primary dysmenorrhea appears to be due to excess production of a prostaglandin (a natural hormonelike chemical) that causes the muscle in the uterine wall to contract. In late pregnancy, this prostaglandin is one factor that triggers labor; contractions help push the baby out. Women with dysmenorrhea experience similar contractions during their periods that produce cramps. Nonsteroidal anti-inflammatory drugs (NSAIDs), such as aspirin, or oral contraceptives are generally the most effective treatment for cramps. Women who exercise regularly seem to experience less dysmenorrhea.

**Contractions and cramps in the uterus**

**Area of pain**
*The pain of primary dysmenorrhea is located in the lower part of the abdomen and sometimes in the lower part of the back. Women do not have to suffer from menstrual pain. Menstrual symptoms can be relieved today by a range of drugs; an understanding doctor will recommend the right one for your needs.*

# DYSMENORRHEA

Dysmenorrhea – painful menstruation – is one of the most common gynecological problems. Again, there are two types of painful menstruation – primary and secondary. Primary dysmenorrhea is menstrual pain that is unrelated to any disease, and it usually develops within the first 2 years of the onset of menstruation. It is a disorder that often runs in families and sometimes disappears or diminishes after the birth of the first child.

In contrast, secondary dysmenorrhea is caused by disorders such as pelvic infection, endometriosis, or intrauterine abnormalities such as fibroid tumors. Effective treatment of pelvic infection or fibroid tumors may eliminate the dysmenorrhea. However, dysmenorrhea caused by endometriosis is often more resistant to treatment.

**Areas of pain**

# ASK YOUR DOCTOR
## MENSTRUAL PROBLEMS

**Q** When one of my friends started taking oral contraceptives, her menstrual pain stopped. Does that always happen?

**A** Some oral contraceptives prevent the release of a mature egg. The "period" that occurs is the result of not taking the pill for 7 days and is not true menstruation; menstrual pain is therefore eliminated. There are no known drawbacks to prolonged oral contraceptive use unless you are a smoker over the age of 35. Use of oral contraceptives can provide two benefits at the same time – relief from cramps and effective contraception.

**Q** I read that you are at risk of iron-deficiency anemia if you have heavy periods. Could you explain more about it?

**A** Anemia is a reduced level of hemoglobin, the oxygen-carrying pigment in the blood. Iron is an essential constituent of hemoglobin. Iron-deficiency anemia can develop in women who shed a lot of menstrual blood, simply because they are losing large amounts of iron and hemoglobin and may not be replacing it in their diet. Your doctor may prescribe iron supplements if anemia has developed.

**Q** For about a week before my menstrual period, I am bloated and achy. Will taking extra vitamins help?

**A** Taking vitamin and mineral supplements, such as vitamin $B_6$, vitamin E, magnesium, and zinc, appears to help some women. However, research has not clearly demonstrated their effectiveness.

# COMFORT AND HYGIENE DURING MENSTRUATION

A daily shower or bath is especially refreshing during your menstrual period. However, the vagina is self-cleansing and douches or antiseptics are not necessary – in fact, using such products may introduce an infection into the vagina or aggravate an infection that is already there. Always (not only during your period) wipe yourself from front to back after going to the toilet to avoid transferring bacteria from the anus into the vulva. Use this same technique when you are washing your genitals. Whether you choose tampons or napkins to contain the menstrual blood loss is entirely up to you.

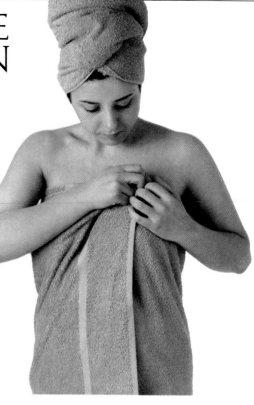

### Sanitary pads
*Sanitary pads are made of absorbent synthetic fibers and wood pulp. The pads are especially convenient for women who menstruate so heavily on some days of their period that tampons cannot absorb all of the flow. A disadvantage of pads is that the menstrual blood is exposed to air and odor may be more of a problem. Change pads at least every 4 to 6 hours.*

### Cleanliness
*Your daily shower or bath during your menstrual period will help you relax. While washing your genital area, do not allow soap to get inside the vagina because it may irritate the tissue.*

### Tampons
*Tampons are made of compressed cotton or rayon material to absorb menstrual blood. They can be safely inserted with a clean finger or with an applicator. Tampons have the advantage of being convenient and inconspicuous. However, because they are used inside the body, it is possible to forget to remove them. Remember to remove one tampon before inserting another; if you feel you must use two at once, make sure you remove them both. See your doctor immediately if you cannot retrieve one that you have inserted. Never use tampons that are impregnated with a chemical, such as a deodorant. These tampons can irritate the vagina and cause serious infections.*

### Vaginal deodorants
*Commercial vaginal deodorant sprays are marketed as products that provide a pleasant odor and mask the natural odor of your body. Use of vaginal deodorant sprays is not recommended because they may cause a chemical inflammation of the vaginal lining, resulting in irritation and discharge. Some women have an allergic reaction to chemicals contained in the sprays.*

**String**

**Applicator**

**Tampon**

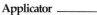

# USING TAMPONS

Today, more and more women use tampons for neatness and freedom from worry about odor. All tampons expand to fit inside your body naturally and comfortably.

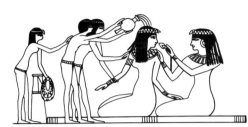

### An ancient solution
*Tampons are nothing new – they have been used throughout the ages in many cultures. Japanese women used paper tampons, Indonesian women made them from vegetable fibers, Romans had woolen tampons, and the Egyptians used papyrus.*

### Using a tampon for the first time
*A young girl inserting a tampon for the first time may need some practice, but she need not worry about losing her virginity. The hymen, the tissue between the internal and external genital organs, has an opening large enough to admit a tampon. Virginity is not defined by the presence of the hymen anyway; a girl is a virgin until she has had sexual intercourse. Tampons made especially for young girls are more slender and may be more comfortable to insert and wear.*

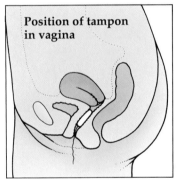

**Position of tampon in vagina**

**WARNING**

Toxic shock syndrome is a rare condition that can occur in menstruating women using tampons. It is caused by toxins (chemicals) produced by a strain of the bacterium *Staphylococcus aureus*. The symptoms of toxic shock syndrome include a sudden, high fever; vomiting; diarrhea; a rash that looks like a sunburn; dizziness; and fainting. Toxic shock syndrome can rapidly progress from flulike symptoms to a serious illness that can be fatal. If you experience any of these symptoms, remove your tampon and contact your doctor immediately. Do not resume using tampons without first talking to your doctor.

### Tampon use and toxic shock syndrome
*The exact role – if any – that tampon use plays in the incidence of toxic shock syndrome is unclear (see WARNING box). About 10 percent of the reported cases of toxic shock syndrome occur in menstruating women using tampons. One possible explanation is that superabsorbent tampons may be left in place for extended periods of time, allowing bacteria to grow in menstrual fluid. To reduce your risk of toxic shock syndrome, change your tampon at least every 4 to 6 hours. You may choose to confine tampon use to the days of heaviest menstrual flow and to use sanitary pads at night.*

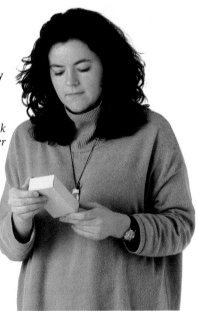

### Tampon absorbency
*The superabsorbent tampons that were implicated in early outbreaks of toxic shock syndrome are no longer available in the US. Today, tampons are manufactured in a range of absorbencies. Use a tampon with the minimum level of absorbency that you need.*

# PREMENSTRUAL SYNDROME

About 70 percent of women notice some changes in the 10 to 14 days before menstrual bleeding starts. For 5 to 10 percent of women, the problem is severe. Common premenstrual symptoms include depression, irritability, headache, fluid retention and weight gain, nausea, breast tenderness, tiredness, and dizziness.

The cause of premenstrual syndrome (PMS) is still unclear. PMS is related to how the levels of estrogen and progesterone affect fluid retention and how the neurotransmitters (chemicals that influence mood) react in the brain during the second half of the cycle.

Treatments are planned to either relieve specific symptoms or to change the hormonal balance in the body. Women are usually advised to exercise regularly and to avoid caffeine, sweets, and salt. These efforts improve general well-being and reduce bloating. Prostaglandin inhibitors such as ibuprofen can alleviate headaches. Progesterone supplements are often prescribed. While most studies have not shown the supplements to be effective, some women report that they help. Oral contraceptives, which suppress ovulation and related hormone secretion, may help some women. Estrogen supplements may be of some benefit. Recent research points toward the use of antidepressant drugs, which increase the supply of the neurotransmitters that affect mood. While there is no cure for PMS, most women can find relief with one or more of these treatments.

**Exercise and PMS**
*Exercise is often helpful in coping with PMS. Choose an exercise routine that you enjoy – swimming or other forms of aerobic exercise such as walking (right) or a relaxation technique such as yoga (left).*

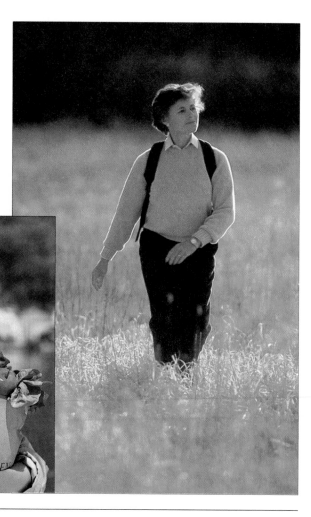

**Changing your diet**
*For some women, dietary changes help reduce or even eliminate the symptoms of PMS. Try to eat plenty of fiber-containing foods, including lots of raw fruit and vegetables. To reduce fluid retention, cut down your sodium intake by avoiding salt and salty foods. Also, avoid sweets.*

# MONITOR YOUR SYMPTOMS
# HEAVY PERIODS

Excessive loss of blood during menstruation is called menorrhagia. Women vary in the amount of blood they lose. If you have excessively heavy periods, talk to your doctor about treatment. Heavy periods can cause iron-deficiency anemia.

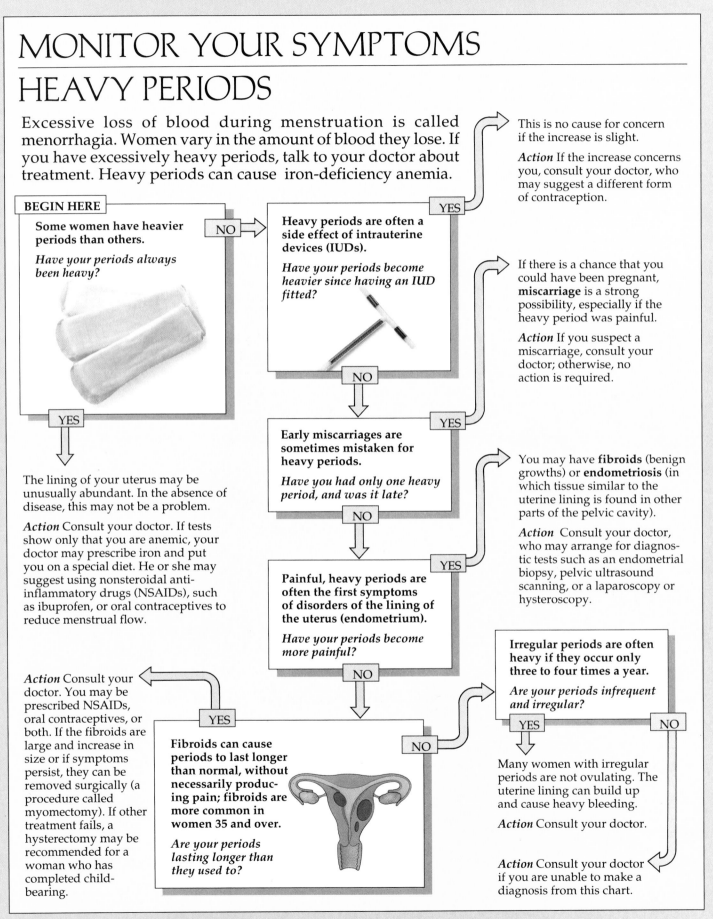

**BEGIN HERE**

**Some women have heavier periods than others.**

*Have your periods always been heavy?*

**NO** →

**Heavy periods are often a side effect of intrauterine devices (IUDs).**

*Have your periods become heavier since having an IUD fitted?*

**YES** →

This is no cause for concern if the increase is slight.

*Action* If the increase concerns you, consult your doctor, who may suggest a different form of contraception.

**NO** ↓

**Early miscarriages are sometimes mistaken for heavy periods.**

*Have you had only one heavy period, and was it late?*

**YES** →

If there is a chance that you could have been pregnant, **miscarriage** is a strong possibility, especially if the heavy period was painful.

*Action* If you suspect a miscarriage, consult your doctor; otherwise, no action is required.

**YES** ↓

The lining of your uterus may be unusually abundant. In the absence of disease, this may not be a problem.

*Action* Consult your doctor. If tests show only that you are anemic, your doctor may prescribe iron and put you on a special diet. He or she may suggest using nonsteroidal anti-inflammatory drugs (NSAIDs), such as ibuprofen, or oral contraceptives to reduce menstrual flow.

**NO** ↓

**Painful, heavy periods are often the first symptoms of disorders of the lining of the uterus (endometrium).**

*Have your periods become more painful?*

**YES** →

You may have **fibroids** (benign growths) or **endometriosis** (in which tissue similar to the uterine lining is found in other parts of the pelvic cavity).

*Action* Consult your doctor, who may arrange for diagnostic tests such as an endometrial biopsy, pelvic ultrasound scanning, or a laparoscopy or hysteroscopy.

**NO** ↓

**Fibroids can cause periods to last longer than normal, without necessarily producing pain; fibroids are more common in women 35 and over.**

*Are your periods lasting longer than they used to?*

**YES** ←

*Action* Consult your doctor. You may be prescribed NSAIDs, oral contraceptives, or both. If the fibroids are large and increase in size or if symptoms persist, they can be removed surgically (a procedure called myomectomy). If other treatment fails, a hysterectomy may be recommended for a woman who has completed childbearing.

**NO** →

**Irregular periods are often heavy if they occur only three to four times a year.**

*Are your periods infrequent and irregular?*

**YES** ↓

Many women with irregular periods are not ovulating. The uterine lining can build up and cause heavy bleeding.

*Action* Consult your doctor.

**NO** ↓

*Action* Consult your doctor if you are unable to make a diagnosis from this chart.

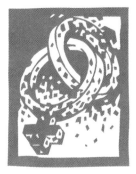

# SEXUALLY TRANSMITTED DISEASES

S EXUALLY TRANSMITTED DISEASES, also called venereal diseases, are infections that are acquired primarily through sexual contact. The organisms responsible for the disease are passed on during intimate contact (especially through oral, genital, or anal intercourse) with a person who has the infection. The incidence of sexually transmitted diseases is increasing rapidly in the US.

Sexually transmitted diseases (STDs) include some of the most common infections in the US. Estimates suggest that about 100,000 American women are made sterile by STDs every year. The organisms that cause the diseases include bacteria, viruses, and other microbes.

## TRANSMISSION AND PREVENTION

We cannot eliminate all of the organisms responsible for STDs but we can avoid them. The organisms that cause STDs can be passed between a woman and her sexual partner via direct genital contact with the vagina, vulva, mouth, or anus or by infectious organisms present in semen or saliva coming into contact with

the moist mucous membrane linings of those parts of a woman's body. Certain infectious organisms (notably HIV – the human immunodeficiency virus that causes AIDS) that are mainly sexually transmitted can also be transmitted in other ways, such as through contact with contaminated blood.

Barrier methods of contraception are recommended for the prevention of many STDs. A condom is effective against most STDs provided the man puts it on his penis before it touches your genital area and removes it after he withdraws. A diaphragm provides some protection against infections of the cervix. To prevent STDs, either method should be used with spermicides that have an antimicrobial action.

### Who is at risk?

You are at increased risk of acquiring an STD if you have unprotected sex with any infected person. A woman is likely to acquire an STD if her partner has it, so fidelity to one partner does not provide complete protection. The more sexual partners you or your partner have, the greater your risk of contracting an STD. STDs can be spread during both homosexual and heterosexual sex. Any break in the lining of the surfaces with which infected genitals come into contact increases the risk of an STD.

**Treatment of infection**
*Most STDs can be cured completely if they are diagnosed early. If you have had sexual contact with anyone who you know or suspect to have an STD or if any unusual symptoms develop, such as sores on the genitals or burning during urination, seek medical advice immediately.*

# AIDS

Acquired immunodeficiency syndrome (AIDS) is a failure of the immune system caused by infection with human immunodeficiency virus (HIV). The AIDS virus is carried in bodily fluids (especially blood and semen). The virus can be transmitted in contaminated blood via transfusion or by sharing needles used to inject drugs of abuse, although many victims contract the disease through sexual intercourse. This dangerous virus was originally thought to be transmitted sexually only among homosexual men, but transmission of the virus among heterosexuals is rapidly increasing. AIDS has not been proved to be transmitted by mosquitoes or by sneezing, coughing, hugging, or sharing food utensils.

HIV infection may be suspected in a person in a high-risk group if he or she has enlargement of the lymph glands or an unexplained weight loss. Testing for HIV involves examining a blood sample for the presence of antibodies to HIV. These antibodies are not found in a person who has only recently been infected with the virus, and anyone considered at risk should have the test again after 6 months. A positive result is confirmed by other tests to remove any margin for error because the most commonly performed test occasionally gives false-positive results. There is no cure for AIDS, but the symptoms and complications of the disease respond to antibiotics, anti-cancer drugs, and antiviral agents. Zidovudine, which is an antiviral drug, has serious side effects, but it slows the progression of AIDS.

## "SAFE" SEX

Safe sex techniques include reducing the number of sexual partners, ideally to one monogamous partner. Partners should use a condom and spermicide for vaginal, oral, and anal intercourse, and ejaculation into the mouth should be avoided. Anal intercourse carries greater risk than vaginal intercourse and should be avoided. HIV carriers should not donate blood or share needles to inject drugs.

## HOW THE AIDS VIRUS AFFECTS THE BODY

The AIDS virus enters the bloodstream of an infected person and weakens the immune system. This leads to AIDS. Individuals with HIV infection may not show symptoms or signs of the disease for several years. These people have antibodies to the virus in their blood and they are called HIV-positive, or carriers. HIV-positive individuals can transmit the virus; to help prevent the spread of the disease, neither they nor their partners should have unprotected sex.

2 HIV (the AIDS virus) attacks and destroys T helper cells. This weakens the immune system and makes it unable to fight off many types of pathogens (harmful organisms).

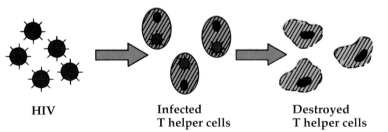

**HIV**  **Infected T helper cells**  **Destroyed T helper cells**

1 Normally, types of white blood cells called T helper cells help to regulate the response of other cells of the immune system in destroying disease-causing organisms (pathogens).

3 Invading harmful organisms can then overwhelm the immune system, rendering the victim susceptible to life-threatening diseases such as pneumonia and Kaposi's sarcoma (a type of cancer). Other infections that are more common or more severe in people with AIDS include herpesvirus infections (such as shingles), tuberculosis, cytomegalovirus infections, and thrush.

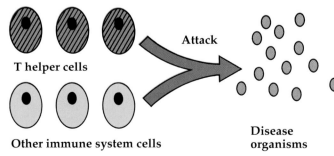

**T helper cells**

**Attack**

**Other immune system cells**

**Disease organisms**

**Overwhelmed immune system cells**

# CHLAMYDIA AND PELVIC INFLAMMATORY DISEASE

Chlamydiae are a group of microorganisms that cause various diseases. In the US, chlamydia is a major cause of genitourinary infection. An estimated 5 to 13 percent of all women in the US have chlamydial infection of the cervix, which is often symptomless. Until recently, chlamydia was regarded as a minor infection. We now know that chlamydia is a major cause of infections of the cervix and urethra and of pelvic inflammatory disease. Pelvic inflammatory disease can cause infertility and recurrent pain.

### The chlamydial organism
*The organism* Chlamydia trachomatis *(see arrows below) was once thought to be a virus because it grows inside the body's cells. It is difficult to detect and grow in a laboratory. Blood tests do not reliably detect it, but special diagnostic tests are now available and are done more frequently as the seriousness of chlamydial infection becomes better known.*

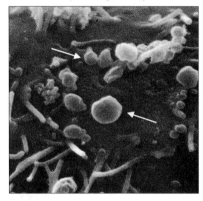

### What are the symptoms of chlamydia?
*Between 10 and 20 days after exposure to the organisms, you may notice pain when you urinate, pain in the lower portion of the abdomen, or possibly a thin vaginal discharge. However, up to 70 percent of women have no symptoms at all. The first sign of a chlamydial infection may be infertility or an ectopic pregnancy (below) caused by inflammation and scarring of the fallopian tubes.*

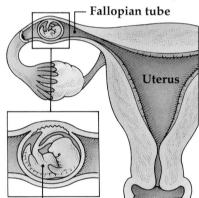

**Fallopian tube**

**Uterus**

**Embryo**

### Can chlamydia be treated?
*Tetracycline (or erythromycin if you are pregnant or allergic to tetracycline) can cure a chlamydial infection, but you and your partner should avoid intercourse until the infection clears up, and all sex partners should be treated. This treatment will not reverse any damage already done to your fallopian tubes.*

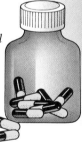

### What is pelvic inflammatory disease?
*Pelvic inflammatory disease is a general term meaning inflammation of the female reproductive organs, especially the uterus, fallopian tubes, and ovaries. The most common cause is infection with chlamydia, but it is also caused by infection with other types of organisms such as mycoplasma (below) and bacteria.*

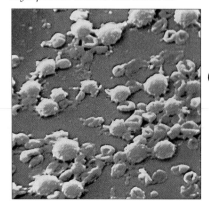

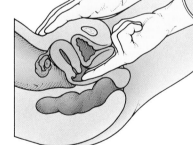

### Who is at risk?
*Any woman who has had multiple sexual partners has an increased risk. The use of an intrauterine device (IUD) also increases the risk slightly; barrier methods, such as condoms, reduce the risk.*

### How is it diagnosed?
*Your doctor will take samples of your vaginal discharge for culture and will perform a bimanual examination (above), including putting gentle pressure on your cervix. This procedure reveals any deep tenderness in the cervix or enlarged, swollen, or pus-filled fallopian tubes and ovaries. The most accurate way to evaluate pelvic inflammatory disease is by laparoscopy, in which the organs are examined through a viewing instrument.*

# WHAT ARE THE SYMPTOMS?

The symptoms of pelvic inflammatory disease may be so mild that you do not notice them. You may experience tiredness, fever, and lack of appetite. In extreme cases, however, the pain may be so intense that you must go to the emergency room. The following symptoms are, singly or together, associated with pelvic inflammatory disease.

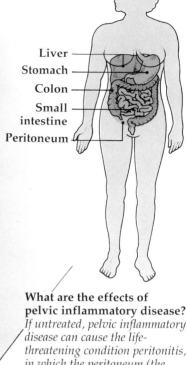

Liver
Stomach
Colon
Small intestine
Peritoneum

**Fever**
*Many women with pelvic inflammatory disease have fever, sweating, and sometimes headache.*

**Location of pain**
*Pelvic inflammatory disease typically causes pain in the same areas of the body where menstrual pain occurs. Common sites include the abdomen, pelvic region, lower part of the back, and legs.*

**Symptoms of chronic pelvic inflammatory disease**
*Chronic pelvic inflammatory disease can be difficult to diagnose because it sometimes causes vague, nonspecific symptoms, including nausea, vomiting, dizziness, fatigue, and abdominal pain.*

**Infected fallopian tube**

**Uterus**

**Normal fallopian tube**

**What are the effects of pelvic inflammatory disease?**
*If untreated, pelvic inflammatory disease can cause the life-threatening condition peritonitis, in which the peritoneum (the membrane that lines the abdominal cavity, see above) becomes inflamed. If not treated early enough, it can permanently damage fallopian tubes, sometimes leading to ectopic (tubal) pregnancy or infertility. It is estimated that one in 10 women with chronic pelvic inflammatory disease will become infertile, the risk increasing with each recurrence of the disease.*

**Reproductive organs**
*Pelvic inflammatory disease affects a woman's reproductive organs, often causing a heavy vaginal discharge, pain or bleeding during or after sexual intercourse, and spotting between periods. It may also cause a burning sensation on urination.*

**How is it usually treated?**
*Antibiotics are prescribed as soon as pelvic inflammatory disease is diagnosed. Tetracycline is often the drug chosen for mild cases because it is effective against chlamydia and most strains of gonorrhea. Once the results of your blood culture are known, you may be switched to a more specific antibiotic. A long course of antibiotics is usually required, and analgesics and anti-inflammatory drugs can relieve the pain. If infection is treated early, there is a strong chance that the bacteria will be eradicated. All recent sexual partners should also be treated.*

**Surgical treatment**
*Antibiotics usually eliminate the active infection of pelvic inflammatory disease, but surgical drainage may be required for large abscesses (pockets of pus). Surgery may be required to open tubes blocked by scar tissue that can form as a result of the disease. If a woman has recurrent episodes, a hysterectomy and removal of the fallopian tubes and ovaries may be recommended.*

95

## GENITAL WARTS

Genital warts are small, firm protuberances that are caused by the human papilloma-virus. A woman can have warts on the inside of her vagina or on her cervix as well as on the skin around her vagina and anus. The incubation period for genital warts can be a few weeks or several months or years. Genital warts may be treated with a topical medication or be painlessly frozen, cauterized, surgically re-moved, or vapor-ized with a laser. Research shows that women exposed to some types of genital warts are at risk of cervical, vaginal, or vulvar cancers. Regular gyneco-logic examination is recommended because these cancers are curable if detected early.

## GONORRHEA

Gonorrhea is a highly infectious disease that is caused by the bacterium *Neisseria gonorrhoeae* and is usually transmitted sexually. Intimate acts such as oral-geni-tal contact may also spread gonorrhea. Children may be exposed as a result of sexual abuse. Children born to infected mothers may acquire gonorrheal oph-thalmia, an eye inflammation that (with-out preventive treatment at birth) may lead to blindness.

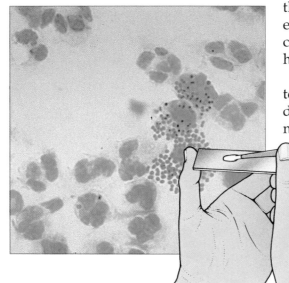

## What happens after infection?

The bacteria that cause gonorrhea spread along the passages of the genital and urinary organs and affect the cervix and urethra. If contact occurs, the anus and throat can be affected. The infection is more likely to persist without symptoms and spread in women than men. If un-treated, it can lead to pelvic inflamma-tory disease (see page 94). Gonorrhea usually attacks the urinary opening, causing a burning sensation on urina-tion. If the cervix is infected, the bacteria cause a copious yellow discharge from the vagina. Gonorrhea seriously threat-ens a pregnancy because the infection can spread via the bloodstream to the heart, brain, liver, and joints.

Gonorrhea is uncommonly treated today with penicillin or tetracycline. The development of resistant bacteria has necessitated the use of other drugs.

**Identifying gonorrhea**
*Many disorders can cause excessive vaginal discharge. Your doctor will try to establish the exact cause by taking a sample of discharge for culture. He or she will also test for antibiotic sensitivity in order to determine what drug to prescribe. The smear is treated with a stain that reveals the gonorrhea bacteria if they are present (far left).*

## HEPATITIS

Hepatitis B and C are viral infections that, before routine blood screening was intro-duced, were often spread via contaminated blood transfusions. These viruses are also transmitted by sexual intercourse, by shared hypodermic needles, or by the passage of blood from mother to fetus. Hepatitis can be transferred by exchange of saliva or exposure to infected secretions such as semen, feces, urine, or blood. Hepatitis B infection may be symptomless or may cause a flulike illness with jaundice. The symp-toms of hepatitis C are usually slightly milder. Both infections can lead to chronic hepatitis and eventually to irreversible liver damage such as cirrhosis or liver cancer.

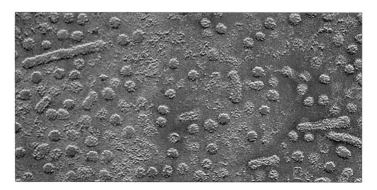

**Hepatitis B infection**
*Hepatitis B virus (above) can persist for years, causing permanent liver damage. Hepatitis is diagnosed by detecting viral particles or antibodies to the virus in the blood. Vaccines are available, but they are usually offered only to those at high risk of infection, such as children born to infected women, drug abusers, male homosexuals, family members of those infected, and health care workers.*

# CASE HISTORY
# UNUSUAL VAGINAL DISCHARGE

TWO WEEKS AGO, Angela noticed that the discharge from her vagina had a foul odor. She tolerated the problem at first, thinking that it would go away without treatment, but the unusual discharge did not disappear. She began to feel pain when she urinated or had sexual intercourse. Angela and her husband are newlyweds, married for only 6 months. Embarrassed about the odor and worried about the pain, Angela made an appointment to see her doctor.

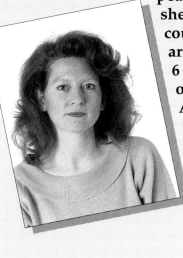

**PERSONAL DETAILS**
**Name** Angela Simpson
**Age** 28
**Occupation** Cosmetologist
**Family** Both of Angela's parents are well.

## MEDICAL BACKGROUND
Angela has always been healthy. She has never had any disease of the genitourinary tract. She has had a satisfying and problem-free sexual relationship with her husband Ron, who seems healthy.

## THE CONSULTATION
The doctor asks Angela to describe her discharge, and she says it is foamy, foul-smelling, and yellow-green. She tells the doctor that it has been this way for the last 2 weeks. The doctor examines a sample of the discharge in his office. He finds *Trichomonas vaginalis* organisms in the sample. No other microorganisms were found in a sample of the discharge that he sent to a laboratory for bacterial culture.

## THE DIAGNOSIS
The doctor tells Angela that she has TRICHOMONIASIS, an infection that is usually sexually transmitted. Be-

cause Ron has been her only sexual partner for more than 2 years, the doctor suggests that he be tested as well. The doctor assures them that trichomoniasis is often symptomless in men. Ron may have had the infec-

**A one-celled parasite**
*Tests on Angela and her husband reveal that they are infected with a protozoal organism,* Trichomonas vaginalis *(right).*

tion for several years without knowing it. Ron is tested that same week and the results confirm that he has trichomoniasis too. The doctor explains to them that Angela has only now exhibited symptoms because, as with many sexually transmitted infections, symptoms usually develop only after repeated exposure.

## THE TREATMENT
Angela and her husband are treated at the same time, to eliminate the possibility of reinfection. If partners are treated at different times, they can continue to pass the infection back and forth – a so-called ping-pong effect. The drug of choice for trichomoniasis is metronidazole, which is taken orally. After the recommended course of 7 to 10 days, Angela's unpleasant discharge ceases and the pain disappears. She and Ron resume their usual loving sexual relationship.

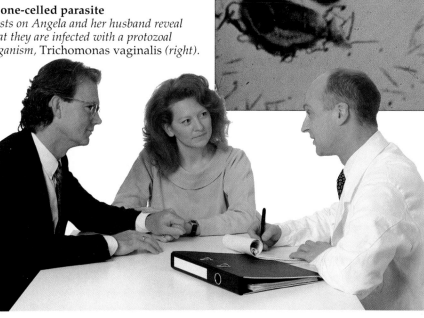

## URETHRITIS

Urethritis is one of the most common diseases caused by sexually transmitted organisms. The term describes inflammation of the urethra caused by a variety of different organisms, but commonly by organisms that inhabit your colon, or by gonococcus or chlamydia. The infection is more common in men and causes a discharge of mucus and pus from the penis. Women may have no symptoms but in most cases experience an increase in frequency of urination, accompanied by a burning sensation. Urethritis is easily treated with antibiotics. Its symptoms and signs should never be ignored because the infection can have serious complications if left untreated. Relapses are common.

# SYPHILIS

Syphilis was once a fatal disease, but it can now be treated with penicillin. The disease is caused by *Treponema pallidum*, a spirochete (spiral bacterium) that penetrates broken skin or mucous membranes in the genitalia, rectum, or mouth during sexual activity. The risk of infection during a single contact with an infected person is about 10 percent. This risk increases with frequency of intercourse with a contagious sexual partner.

During the late 1980s, an alarming 25 percent increase in syphilis in the US was linked to use of illicit drugs, especially crack, an inexpensive, smokable form of cocaine. Crack is highly addictive and it enhances sexual desire. Disadvantaged women addicts frequently turn to prostitution to pay for the drug.

Because of the link between crack, sex, and prostitution, many of these women become pregnant and pass syphilis on to their children. Congenital syphilis in infants had become rare, but the incidence is rising in some city populations in the US. In all racial groups, increases were greater for women than for men.

## The stages of syphilis

The first stage of syphilis is the appearance of a painless, hard, ulcerated sore called a chancre on the genitals or cervix or in the anus or mouth. This sore heals in 6 to 10 weeks.

In the second stage of syphilis, which occurs 6 weeks to 6 months after the appearance of the primary chancre, the bacteria enter the bloodstream and cause lymph gland enlargement and a widespread rash on the body, palms, and mucous membranes. Syphilitic warts may appear on the genitals. The person is highly infectious while in this second stage, which lasts from 2 to 6 weeks.

A long latent period then occurs in which there are no symptoms. By the third stage, the syphilis bacteria can attack any organ. Even at this stage, syphilis can be cured with penicillin, but organ damage cannot be reversed.

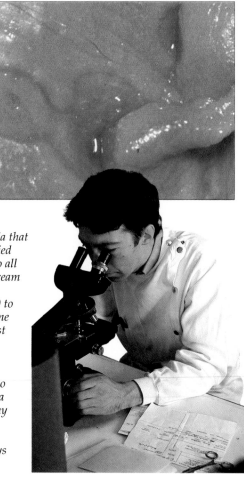

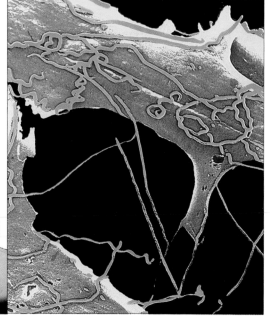

**Identifying syphilis**
*Once inside the body, the bacteria that cause syphilis (far right, magnified 5,000 times) pass very quickly to all parts of the body via the bloodstream and the lymphatic system. The incubation period varies from 10 to 90 days, and it may be a long time before the development of the first syphilitic sore (above). To diagnose syphilis, a microscope (right) is used to identify the bacteria scraped from a sore. If no sore is present, a test is done on a sample. A positive test result may not be obtained until 4 weeks after the appearance of the first sore. Blood test results are always positive in secondary syphilis.*

## PUBIC LICE

Pubic lice ("crabs") are small wingless insects that infest pubic hair and feed on blood. You can acquire pubic lice (below, magnified 45 times) from close body contact with a person who is infested. The main symptom is severe itching. Scratching the affected area can transmit the lice to other parts of the body. The lice are

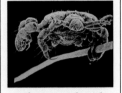

easily treated with a shampoo containing lindane, pyrethrins, or permethrin. Sexual partners should also be treated.

# GENITAL HERPES

Genital herpes is a viral condition that causes a painful rash. The main danger of herpes is its tendency to increase susceptibility to other sexually transmitted diseases (such as AIDS), in part because of the presence of open sores. The first attack of herpes is usually the most severe. Then the virus lies dormant in the roots of the spinal nerves. At this time there are no symptoms but the person may be capable of infecting others. Recurrent attacks are common; sexual activity should be avoided completely until the symptoms have disappeared (condoms should be used even when symptoms are absent). The virus that causes genital herpes is closely related to the virus that causes oral herpes (cold sores).

The best treatment for herpes is to obtain as much rest as possible and keep the sores clean and dry. Improvement in symptoms has been achieved with the antiviral drug acyclovir. The sores can be cleared up rapidly and, if the attacks are frequent, the drug can be taken on a long-term basis to prevent recurrence. If a pregnant woman has an attack of genital herpes when her baby is due, a cesarean section is done to prevent the baby from becoming infected during vaginal delivery.

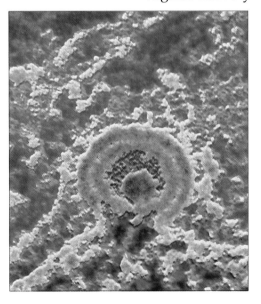

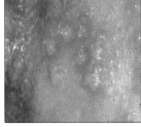

**Herpes simplex virus**
*Genital herpes is caused by the virus herpes simplex 2 (left, magnified 75,500 times). Usually a few days after sexual contact with a person who has active sores, tiny blisters (above) appear on the vulva, penis, or around the anus. These blisters burst and form painful sores.*

# ASK YOUR DOCTOR
# SEXUALLY TRANS-MITTED DISEASES

**Q** **I have had a vaginal discharge for the last few days. Could this mean that I have a sexually transmitted disease?**

**A** Not necessarily. There are a number of circumstances in which a vaginal discharge is normal. A discharge is more common in pregnancy and toward the end of a menstrual cycle. However, if your discharge is creamy or cheesy-looking, is more copious than usual, or has an offensive odor, it is likely to be caused by an infection – which may or may not have been sexually transmitted. Talk to your doctor about your symptoms. Such infections are easily treated once the causative organism has been diagnosed.

**Q** **Can I get a sexually transmitted disease from a towel or toilet seat that has been in contact with an infected person?**

**A** It is highly unlikely that you could acquire a sexually transmitted disease from such a source. The organisms that cause most sexually transmitted diseases are very fragile and cannot live outside the human body for long.

**Q** **I have read that taking oral contraceptives will protect me from getting pelvic inflammatory disease. Is this really true?**

**A** Studies suggest that some oral contraceptives may protect against pelvic inflammatory disease, but don't rely on oral contraceptives alone to protect you. Other preventive measures include limiting the number of your sexual partners and always using condoms.

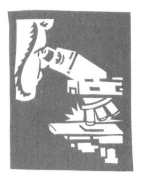

# UTERINE, OVARIAN, AND VAGINAL DISORDERS

**M**ANY OF THE PROBLEMS that women discuss with their doctors are gynecological – that is, they involve some aspect of the reproductive system. A woman may want to ask about a common symptom such as menstrual pain or more serious concerns such as abnormal bleeding. She may routinely call to schedule a general checkup and cervical (Pap) smear.

You can learn the most from your doctor if you volunteer information about your symptoms and ask all the questions you need to understand your diagnosis and treatment. You may wish to take notes on your doctor's explanations and instructions. No aspect of your body's function is too trivial to discuss.

## ENDOMETRIAL POLYPS

Endometrial polyps are benign growths that protrude into the uterine cavity from the inner lining of the uterine wall. Polyps can occur at any age, but they develop most frequently in the 10 years before the menopause. They can cause cramping, irregular periods, and, if they protrude through the cervix, bleeding after intercourse. Polyps are often removed by cautery. If the polyps are particularly large or numerous, dilatation and curettage (D and C) or removal through a hysteroscope may be required (see SURGICAL PROCEDURES on page 101).

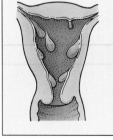

## DISORDERS OF THE UTERUS

The primary function of the uterus is to provide a good environment for a growing embryo and fetus. Each month, the lining of the uterus thickens in preparation for the implantation of a fertilized egg. If conception does not occur, this lining is shed, forming the menstrual flow. Disorders of the menstrual cycle are discussed in MENSTRUAL PROBLEMS on page 86. Other uterine disorders that can occur include fibroids, polyps, cancer, endometriosis, and prolapse.

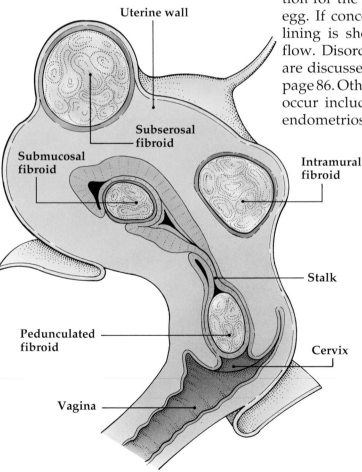

Uterine wall

Subserosal fibroid

Submucosal fibroid

Intramural fibroid

Stalk

Pedunculated fibroid

Cervix

Vagina

**What are fibroids?**
*Fibroids are benign tumors of the uterus composed of fibrous tissue and muscle. They form during a woman's fertile years and usually shrink or stop growing after the menopause. Although their cause is unknown, their growth seems to be related to estrogen production. A woman often has multiple fibroids that may vary in size from the size of a seed to large tumors that fill the abdomen (left). The symptoms that fibroids cause vary depending on their site, which can be just under the inner surface (submucosal fibroids), within the muscular tissue (intramural fibroids), just under the outer surface of the wall of the uterus (subserosal fibroids), or on a stalk (pedunculated fibroids).*

## Fibroids

The uterine fibroid (leiomyoma) is the most common type of tumor to grow in the human body. Approximately one in five women over 35 will have fibroids. These growths are benign (noncancerous) tumors and are often small and symptomless. A heavy menstrual flow is the most common problem women experience with fibroids that grow just under the uterine lining. Large fibroids can also cause abdominal discomfort, back pain, or frequent urination if they press on the bladder.

Most fibroids do not require treatment. Surgery may be advisable if the fibroids are causing troublesome symptoms. A surgeon will either remove just the fibroids (myomectomy) or remove the uterus (hysterectomy). Myomectomy is done if the woman plans to have children. Hysterectomy may be performed less frequently today because alternate medical and surgical treatments for fibroids have been developed.

## Endometrial cancer

About 33,000 new cases of cancer of the endometrium are diagnosed in the US every year. The cancer usually occurs in postmenopausal women and develops more frequently in women who are obese or diabetic, have high blood pressure, have never conceived, or have had a delayed menopause. Irregular bleeding is the most common symptom. Any woman who experiences vaginal bleeding after the menopause should consult a doctor without delay.

Hysterectomy with removal of lymph glands is the most common treatment for endometrial cancer. Radiation therapy, chemotherapy, or hormone therapy may also be required for some women. Because endometrial cancer causes irregular bleeding, doctors can sometimes diagnose the condition early and cure it; 80 percent of all women with endometrial cancer are alive and well 5 years after treatment.

# SURGICAL PROCEDURES
# DILATATION AND CURETTAGE

DILATATION AND curettage (D and C) is a common gynecological operation. It is a procedure used to assess the condition of the endometrium (the lining of the uterus) when a woman has reported abnormal uterine bleeding. A doctor often performs a D and C with the aid of a hysteroscope (an optical instrument) that he or she passes through your cervix to view the inside of your uterus directly. The procedure can confirm or exclude a diagnosis of polyps, fibroids, hyperplasia (thickening of the uterine lining), or cancer. It may provide temporary relief from heavy bleeding, but the D and C does not treat the underlying cause, which is usually hormonal. While D and C is most often a diagnostic tool, it can be done therapeutically to remove a polyp or tissue remaining after a miscarriage. D and C is usually performed while the woman is under general anesthesia. It is normal to experience bleeding for several days afterward.

1 The opening of the cervix is gently dilated (enlarged) by inserting a series of progressively wider rods (dilators).

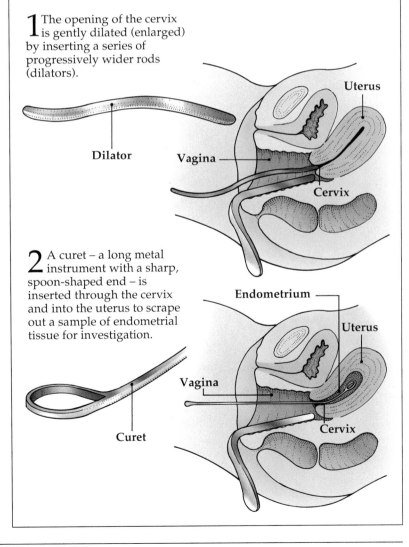

2 A curet – a long metal instrument with a sharp, spoon-shaped end – is inserted through the cervix and into the uterus to scrape out a sample of endometrial tissue for investigation.

# CERVICAL DISORDERS

The cervix, or neck of the uterus, is composed mainly of muscle and fibrous tissue. It forms a passage for menstrual flow out of the uterus and allows sperm to enter the upper reproductive tract. It remains firmly closed during pregnancy to hold the growing fetus within the uterus. The cervix extends into the vagina. Your doctor can feel it and, using a speculum, can see it during vaginal examination. Disorders of the cervix include eversion, polyps, abnormal (precancerous) cell changes, cancer, cervical incompetence (see MISCARRIAGE on page 23), cervicitis, and infections (see SEXUALLY TRANSMITTED DISEASES on page 92).

### Cervical eversion
*Cervical eversion (right) is a normal condition in many women and rarely needs treatment. It occurs when mucus-producing cells, similar to those usually found only inside the cervical canal, form a layer on the outer surface of the cervix (the cervical os). These cells result in a tendency to bleed and occasionally cause heavy vaginal discharge. Cervical eversion occurs most often as a result of pregnancy or long-term use of oral contraceptives and appears to be caused by hormonal changes.*

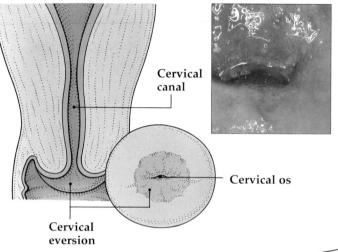

**Cervical canal**

**Cervical os**

**Cervical eversion**

### Cervicitis
*Cervicitis (left) is inflammation with or without infection of the cervix. It is often related to common vaginal infections or sexually transmitted diseases including pelvic inflammatory disease. It can also result from an infection after childbirth or insertion of an intrauterine device (IUD). Symptoms include increased vaginal discharge, pain during intercourse, aching in the lower part of the abdomen, fever, and the urge to urinate more often. If left untreated, chronic cervicitis can cause infertility.*

## CERVICAL CELL CHANGE AND CANCER

Cervical intraepithelial neoplasia (CIN), or cervical dysplasia, consists of cell changes on the surface of the cervix that are abnormal but not yet cancerous. Many mild cases of cervical intraepithelial neoplasia spontaneously revert back to normal. However, if it is not treated, cervical cancer develops in some cases; early diagnosis is extremely important. Your doctor checks for cervical cell changes by doing a cervical (Pap) smear. He or she passes a small spatula into your vagina through a speculum and scrapes cells from your cervical canal. The cells are smeared onto a glass slide (right) and sent to a laboratory to be examined under a microscope.

**Slide**

**Spatula**

### "Precancerous" changes
*Abnormal changes in cervical cells are usually graded according to their severity. CIN1 is mild dysplasia, CIN2 is moderate dysplasia, and CIN3 is severe dysplasia. Views of each of these changes are shown at right.*

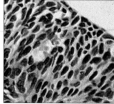

**Normal cells**

**CIN1 changes**

**CIN2 changes**

**CIN3 changes**

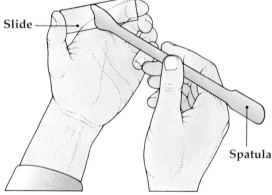

**Cancer cells**

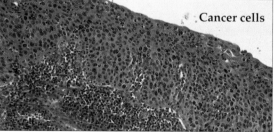

### Cervical cancer
*Cervical cancer (shown above) is the most commonly occurring cancer of the female reproductive tract. The most frequent symptoms are abnormal bleeding or vaginal discharge. Doctors can treat the cancer with either surgery (hysterectomy) or radiation therapy. The cure rate for early stages of cervical cancer is more than 80 percent.*

# DIAGNOSING CERVICAL CHANGES

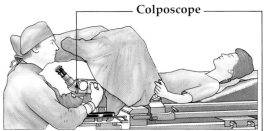

Colposcope

## Colposcopy
If any abnormalities are found in your cervical (Pap) smear, further investigation by colposcopy is usually required. A colposcope (above and right) is an illuminating and magnifying optical instrument that enables your doctor to directly examine your cervix in more detail. Biopsy instruments may be inserted through a speculum.

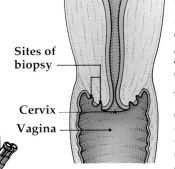

**Biopsy**
During colposcopy, the doctor removes a tiny piece of tissue from abnormal-looking areas of your cervix for further examination. This biopsy (left) is done with sharp, scissorlike forceps. It can be performed with or without local anesthesia.

Sites of biopsy

Cervix

Vagina

## Cone biopsy
If your doctor suspects that cells lying below the surface of your cervix are abnormal, he or she will do a cone biopsy (right). This procedure involves removing a cone-shaped section of tissue from your cervix for further investigation. The operation can be done with either a laser or a scalpel, and it may be performed with local anesthesia. Cone biopsy may also be used to remove cells that have been found to be abnormal.

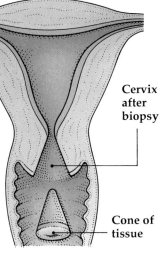

Cervix after biopsy

Cone of tissue

# TREATING CERVICAL CHANGES

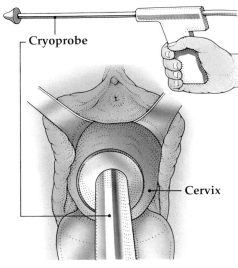

Cryoprobe

Cervix

## Cryocautery
Cryocautery is a procedure that freezes abnormal cervical tissue to destroy it. Liquid nitrogen is released from a tank into an instrument called a cryoprobe (above). Cryocautery works to a depth of only 3 to 4 millimeters so it is unsuitable if the doctor suspects underlying abnormalities. The procedure may cause bleeding and a watery discharge for 2 to 3 weeks after it has been performed.

## Laser treatment
A laser is a device that produces a concentrated beam of light radiation (below). This beam can be used to destroy abnormal cervical cells by vaporizing the water that makes up most of the cells. Laser treatment can be controlled precisely to destroy any abnormal tissue. The procedure is performed after the woman has been given a local anesthetic. Healing generally takes place quickly with few complications.

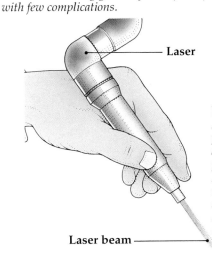

Laser

Laser beam

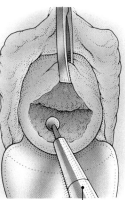

Diathermy probe

## Diathermy
Abnormal cervical cells are destroyed by passing an electric current through the affected area with a probe (above). The patient must be under a general anesthetic. Another type of diathermy passes current through a loop and removes rather than destroys abnormal tissue. This type of diathermy can be performed quickly with the use of a local anesthetic.

# Endometriosis

Endometriosis is a condition in which fragments of tissue that resemble and behave like tissue from the endometrium (the lining of the uterus) grow in other parts of the body, usually in the pelvic area. It is more common among white women and women who have not had children and usually occurs between the ages of 30 and 40. Endometriotic growths respond to the monthly variations in a woman's hormone levels, and they grow and bleed during each menstrual cycle as if they were in the uterus. Unlike menstrual flow, this blood cannot leave the body and the accumulation of blood can lead to inflammation and pain.

Endometriosis may cause painful, heavy periods; discomfort during intercourse; pain in the pelvis and back; and painful or bloody bowel movements or urination. It is also a cause of infertility. About 30 to 40 percent of women with endometriosis are infertile.

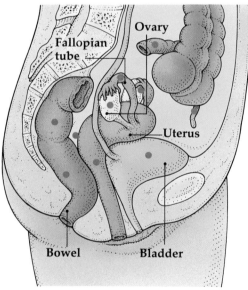

● **Possible sites of endometriosis**

### Treating endometriosis
*Endometriotic growths usually form in the pelvic area. They may grow on the outside of the uterus or on the ovaries, bladder, bowel, or fallopian tubes. To diagnose the condition, your doctor will use an instrument called a laparoscope (see page 108). Endometriosis can be treated with hormonal therapy, surgery, or a combination of both. Surgery with electrocauterization or laser often can be done through the laparoscope.*

# UTERINE PROLAPSE

A prolapsed uterus is displaced from its normal position and sags down into or even out of the vagina. Prolapse occurs when the ligaments holding the uterus in place are stretched by pregnancy and childbirth or are weakened after the menopause. A prolapse may be made worse by a chronic cough, constipation, obesity, or strenuous physical activity. Uterine prolapse may occur with prolapse of the bladder, urethra, or rectum, conditions in which the bladder, urethral wall, or rectal wall bulge into the vaginal wall. Depending on the degree of prolapse, you may have a heavy sensation in your vagina of "something coming down."

**Normal position of uterus**

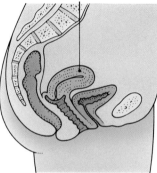

**Prolapsed uterus**

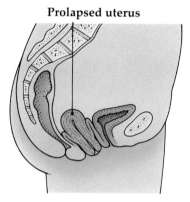

**Supported uterus**

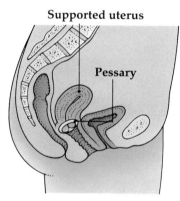

### Treating a prolapse
*For postmenopausal women, hormone replacement therapy will increase the blood supply to the pelvis and may strengthen supportive tissues. If symptoms of prolapse occur, you can have a pessary inserted into your vagina (left). A pessary is a rubber device that fits around the cervix and helps support the uterus. If you cannot wear a pessary, you can have an operation to repair stretched tissues or a hysterectomy.*

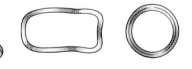

**Types of vaginal pessaries**

### Preventing a prolapse
*Your risk of uterine prolapse is decreased if you do pelvic floor exercises after childbirth (see page 119) and consume large quantities of fiber and fluid to prevent constipation (right). You should also avoid gaining weight, smoking cigarettes (because it can cause a chronic cough), and heavy lifting.*

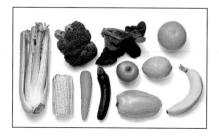

## OVARIAN DISORDERS

The occurrence of tumors is the main problem associated with the ovaries. Ovarian tumors can be benign or malignant and solid or cystic (filled with fluid). Small tumors often cause no symptoms. Symptoms of larger tumors include a swollen abdomen, constipation, incontinence, and abdominal pain.

### Ovarian cysts

Ovarian cysts are fluid-filled tumors that are usually benign. They can occur at any age but are most common in women in their 40s. Once your doctor has felt a tumor during an examination, he or she often uses ultrasound scanning to confirm the diagnosis. Complications of cysts include rupture, bleeding into the cyst, or twisting (torsion) of the cystic ovary, which interrupts its blood supply.

Removal of a cyst by open surgery or laparoscopic surgery while the patient is under a general anesthetic is usually necessary if the cyst is causing symptoms or is larger than 2 inches in diameter. For younger women, only the cyst is removed and the surgeon tries to conserve any unaffected part of the ovary. For women

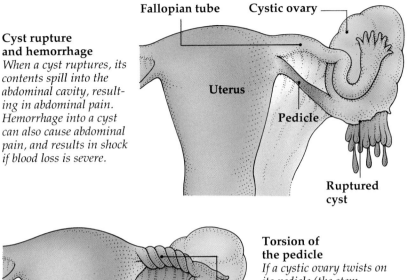

**Fallopian tube**  **Cystic ovary**

**Uterus**

**Pedicle**

**Ruptured cyst**

**Cyst rupture and hemorrhage**
*When a cyst ruptures, its contents spill into the abdominal cavity, resulting in abdominal pain. Hemorrhage into a cyst can also cause abdominal pain, and results in shock if blood loss is severe.*

**Torsion of the pedicle**
*If a cystic ovary twists on its pedicle (the stem through which it receives its blood supply), it causes acute pain and other symptoms; surgery may be required.*

**Twisted fallopian tube and pedicle**

**Polycystic ovaries**
*Ovaries that are polycystic are enlarged with multiple small cysts (below left). Polycystic ovaries cause hormonal imbalances that may result in irregular periods, obesity, growth of body hair, and infertility. Treatment usually consists of drug therapy to regulate hormone levels or to stimulate ovulation in a woman who wants to become pregnant.*

who have completed their families, doctors may remove one or both ovaries, and sometimes the uterus as well, to prevent spread of disease if the cyst turns out to be malignant. About 40 percent of ovarian cysts that occur in women over 40 exhibit some malignancy.

### Ovarian cancer

Although less common than cancers of the uterus and cervix, ovarian cancer kills more women than the other two types combined. Because ovarian cancer tends not to cause symptoms, it is often not diagnosed until the disease is advanced. Ovarian cancer is most common in women in their 50s and 60s.

Ultrasound can be used to evaluate an enlarged ovary detected by physical examination and to help detect malignancy. The primary treatment is surgery, but chemotherapy or radiation therapy is often required. The overall prognosis is poor. The 5-year survival rate is only about 35 to 40 percent.

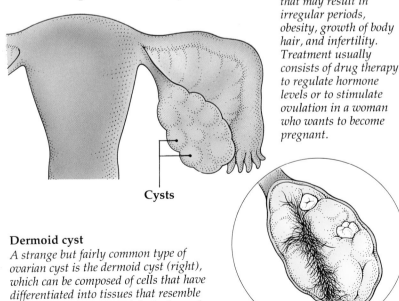

**Cysts**

**Dermoid cyst**
*A strange but fairly common type of ovarian cyst is the dermoid cyst (right), which can be composed of cells that have differentiated into tissues that resemble tissue from other parts of the body, such as the skin, hair, and teeth.*

# SURGICAL PROCEDURES
# HYSTERECTOMY

**H**YSTERECTOMY, **removal of the uterus, is one of the most frequently performed operations in the US. The procedure can be done vaginally or abdominally. The operation may be done for valid reasons such as cancer in the reproductive tract or uncontrolled bleeding. However, in the US, 25 percent of women over 50 have had a hysterectomy, often for minor reasons and sometimes simply because their families are complete. Many doctors now consider some of these operations unnecessary.**

---

### WARNING

A hysterectomy is a major operation – both a woman and her doctor should carefully consider the decision to undertake the procedure. If you are advised to have a hysterectomy, get a second opinion. As with the removal of any other abdominal organ, the procedure poses the risk of complications, such as infection of the incision, bladder, or chest; hemorrhage; and thrombosis (blood clotting). About one woman in every thousand dies as a result of the operation. If you are having the operation before the menopause and your ovaries are left intact, you may still experience some symptoms of the menstrual cycle, but without cramping or bleeding. If your ovaries are removed, you will experience menopausal symptoms and may be given hormone replacement therapy.

---

### Types of hysterectomy
*A hysterectomy can be subtotal (removal of the body of the uterus only, leaving the cervix), an operation almost never performed today; total (removal of the uterus including the cervix); or radical (removal of the uterus, cervix, surrounding tissue, lymph glands, part of the vagina, and sometimes the fallopian tubes and ovaries).*

**Subtotal hysterectomy**

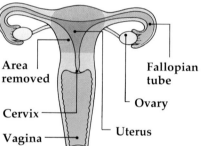

Area removed
Fallopian tube
Ovary
Cervix
Uterus
Vagina

**Total hysterectomy**

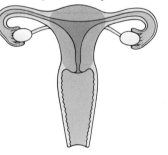

**Radical hysterectomy**

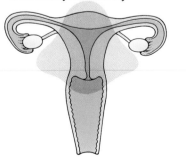

### VAGINAL HYSTERECTOMY
Some doctors may recommend that your uterus be removed vaginally if it is not swollen by disease. Recovery from a vaginal hysterectomy may be quicker and may cause less discomfort because there is no abdominal incision. The operation is often done in conjunction with repair of the vaginal walls if they have been affected by prolapse.

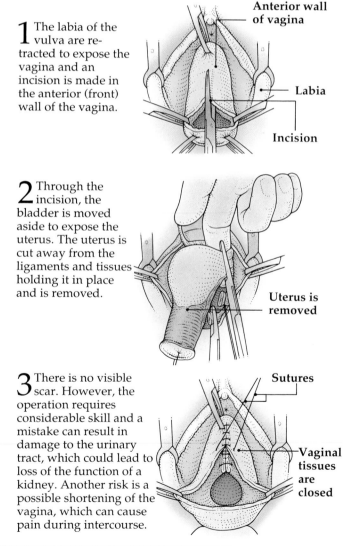

1 The labia of the vulva are retracted to expose the vagina and an incision is made in the anterior (front) wall of the vagina.

Anterior wall of vagina
Labia
Incision

2 Through the incision, the bladder is moved aside to expose the uterus. The uterus is cut away from the ligaments and tissues holding it in place and is removed.

Uterus is removed

3 There is no visible scar. However, the operation requires considerable skill and a mistake can result in damage to the urinary tract, which could lead to loss of the function of a kidney. Another risk is a possible shortening of the vagina, which can cause pain during intercourse.

Sutures
Vaginal tissues are closed

## ABDOMINAL HYSTERECTOMY

If your uterus is enlarged or cancerous or if your ovaries also need to be removed, an abdominal incision is necessary to perform a hysterectomy.

**1** An incision into your abdomen is made either horizontally along the upper pubic hairline or vertically between the navel and pubic hair. A horizontal incision heals quickly and any scar is hidden by the pubic hairline.

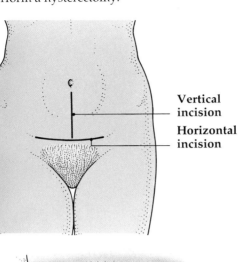

**Vertical incision**

**Horizontal incision**

**2** The uterus is exposed and cut free from the ligaments and other tissues holding it in place. If necessary, the ovaries and fallopian tubes are detached and removed.

**Ligament and fallopian tube are cut**

**Uterus**

**3** The cervix is freed from the bladder, and the cervix and uterus are cut away from the vaginal wall and removed.

**Cervix**

**Uterus**

**Vaginal opening**

## AFTER YOUR HYSTERECTOMY

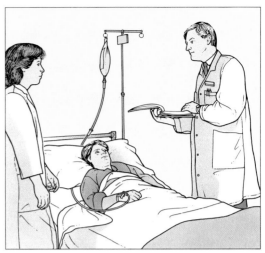

**Recovering in the hospital**
*Most women undergoing a hysterectomy can expect to be in the hospital for a few days. For a day or two after the operation, it is common to have a urinary catheter (tube) inserted into your bladder to help you empty it. Occasionally, a drain is placed in the abdominal incision to prevent the collection of blood under your skin. You are also given fluids intravenously for the first day or two (above).*

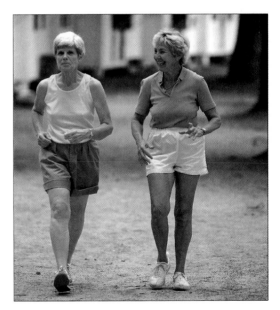

**Recuperating at home**
*Once home from the hospital, you should be careful not to overstrain yourself. Driving may be unwise for at least 2 weeks because postoperative painkillers may slow your reaction time and pain in the lower part of your abdomen and the upper part of your thighs might interfere with your driving skills. Refrain from sexual intercourse until your doctor has examined you (usually 4 to 6 weeks after the operation). Walking is an excellent exercise to help you recover your strength and energy. Try walking for 10 minutes every day and work up to 30 to 45 minutes.*

# VAGINAL AND VULVAL PROBLEMS

Common problems associated with the vaginal and vulval (external) areas include infection, atrophy (thinning or shrinking), and dystrophy (disrupted cellular development or activity).

## Vaginal infections

The most common causes of vaginitis (vaginal inflammation) are the fungus *Candida albicans*, the parasite *Trichomonas vaginalis*, and several bacteria. Most women have one or more of these infections (which are not the result of poor hygiene) at some time. Some infections, such as those produced by chlamydia, may be sexually transmitted (see SEXUALLY TRANSMITTED DISEASES on page 92). The signs of vaginal infection include a heavy or foul-smelling discharge, discomfort, and itching. Treatment is usually effective. Depending on what type of organism is causing the infection, your doctor may recommend an antibacterial, antibiotic, or antifungal agent. One antifungal agent is now available without a prescription.

## Atrophy and dystrophy

The drop in your estrogen level that occurs after the menopause can cause atrophy (thinning and shrinking) of the vulva and vagina (see MENOPAUSAL PROBLEMS on page 124). This condition should respond to hormone therapy; a lack of response suggests that a vulval dystrophy (disrupted tissue growth) may be present. All types of dystrophy cause itching and discomfort, and the skin may be thin or thickened, red or white, and occasionally ulcerated. To diagnose the disorder, a doctor must perform a biopsy. Steroid creams are usually prescribed for treatment, but some women do not respond well and may need some skin removed from their vulva.

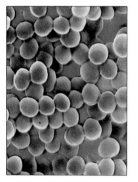

**Vaginitis**
*Infection with the fungus* Candida albicans *(left, magnified 3,000 times) causes a discharge that looks something like cottage cheese. This infection occurs most often in pregnant women, in women taking antibiotics or oral contraceptives, and in women with diabetes.*

**VULVAL CANCER**
Cancer of the vulva is uncommon and occurs mainly in women over 60. Some cases are preceded by noticeable symptoms. The most common symptoms are a lump or ulcer or persistent itching and discomfort. A biopsy is required to diagnose vulval cancer. The diseased areas are surgically removed. Treatment is usually effective, particularly if the disease is diagnosed early. It is important not to delay consulting your doctor if you notice symptoms.

## LAPAROSCOPIC SURGERY

The laparoscope is an optical instrument that allows a surgeon to view the inside of your abdomen through a small incision, usually made in your navel. The laparoscope can be used to diagnose pelvic inflammatory disease, to investigate ectopic pregnancy, to assess the fallopian tubes in cases of infertility, and to perform some surgical procedures. Tubal ligation, removal of an ovarian cyst, removal of an ectopic pregnancy, electrocautery or laser treatment of endometriosis, and removal of fibroids can all be performed using instruments passed through the laparoscope. The advantages of laparoscopic surgery are that you do not need to stay in the hospital for long and there is less discomfort after the operation.

**The laparoscope**
*The laparoscope has a fiberoptic light source and a range of wide-angle lenses at the end. It is inserted in your abdomen to give the surgeon a direct view of the pelvic organs. The surgeon can view the field on a television monitor.*

# CASE HISTORY
# AN UNSUSPECTED PROBLEM

Diane and her fiancé were looking forward to raising a family. They had often discussed how they would manage their professional lives and their future roles as parents. Diane recently scheduled an appointment with her gynecologist for her regular checkup. At her last appointment 2 years ago the gynecological examination had revealed no problems, and the results of the cervical (Pap) smear had been normal.

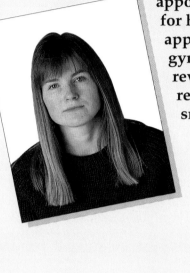

**PERSONAL DETAILS**
**Name** Diane Walters
**Age** 28
**Occupation** Salesperson
**Family** Diane's mother is well. Her father suffers from angina.

## MEDICAL BACKGROUND
Apart from breaking her left arm as a child, Diane has always enjoyed good health. She is a vegetarian and a nonsmoker. Her periods are regular and free of pain or discomfort.

## THE CONSULTATION
During the consultation, the gynecologist asks Diane a series of questions about her health. She tells him that she has not noticed any unusual symptoms. She also informs him of her upcoming marriage. The gynecologist then examines Diane. He performs a cervical (Pap) smear followed by a manual examination. During the latter, he discovers a swelling of about 3 inches in diameter in Diane's left ovary. He suspects this is a benign cyst resulting from excessive enlargement of a follicle in the ovary. Because oral contraceptives sometimes cause this type of cyst to shrink without further treatment, the gynecologist pre-

scribes treatment with oral contraceptives. He asks Diane to return in 6 weeks to see if the treatment has been successful.

## THE DIAGNOSIS
When Diane returns for her follow-up examination, she is disappointed to learn that her ovarian swelling has not disappeared and is, in fact,

slightly larger than before. The gynecologist arranges for her to have a pelvic ultrasound examination the same day. The investigation reveals a fluid-filled swelling in her left ovary, confirming that Diane has developed an OVARIAN CYST.

## THE TREATMENT
The gynecologist advises Diane that the cyst should be surgically removed for two reasons. First, he explains that complications may develop, possibly causing damage to the ovary. Second, he tells Diane that there is a slight possibility of cancer, although this is very unlikely at her age. A few days later, Diane comes to the hospital's outpatient department for laparoscopic surgery (see page 108). The cyst is sent to the pathology laboratory for examination under a microscope.

## THE OUTCOME
Three days after the operation, the gynecologist tells Diane that the pathology report confirms that the cyst was benign. Diane is relieved, but still concerned that her chances of having children may be reduced. Her gynecologist reassures her that her ovary is not damaged and her ability to conceive is unimpaired.

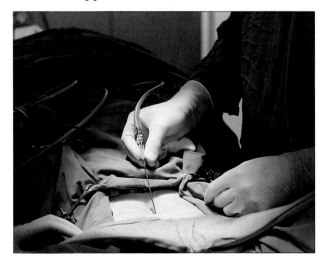

**Removing the cyst**
*During surgery, the gynecologist removes the entire cyst from Diane's ovary. He is pleased to see that most of the organ appears to be unaffected.*

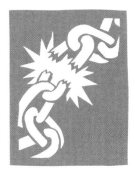

# INFERTILITY

**I**NFERTILITY WAS ONCE thought to be a woman's problem. Today we know that the numbers of infertile men and women are about equal. Doctors can now determine the causes of a couple's infertility 85 to 95 percent of the time. Even in those cases where the causes remain unclear, ingenious techniques are available to help many couples or individuals have a child.

A variety of problems can cause a couple to be unable to conceive. The first step in the management of infertility is a comprehensive investigation to discover whether a definite cause can be found. Some of the causes and investigations of female fertility problems are discussed in SITES OF FEMALE INFERTILITY on page 111. See page 112 for discussions of MALE INFERTILITY and UNEXPLAINED INFERTILITY.

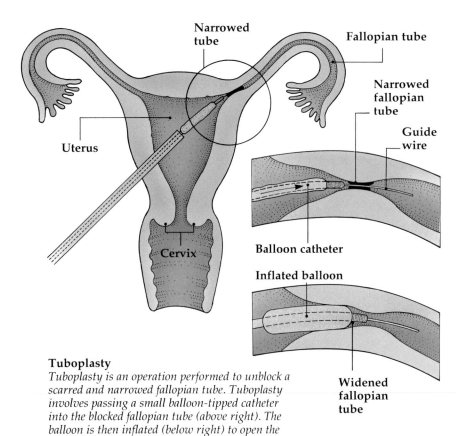

**Tuboplasty**
*Tuboplasty is an operation performed to unblock a scarred and narrowed fallopian tube. Tuboplasty involves passing a small balloon-tipped catheter into the blocked fallopian tube (above right). The balloon is then inflated (below right) to open the damaged tube and create a passage for unfertilized eggs to move from the ovary through the fallopian tube to be fertilized. The balloon is then deflated and the catheter withdrawn.*

## TREATMENTS FOR FEMALE INFERTILITY

About 40 percent of all fertility problems are caused by factors affecting the female partner. When the cause of infertility has been established, a doctor tries either to cure the underlying disorder so that conception is possible or, if the condition is untreatable, he or she will discuss the appropriate artificial methods of achieving pregnancy.

### Treatments for anovulation

In developed countries, the most common cause of anovulation (absence of egg production) is excessive weight loss, sometimes the result of depression. Anovulation can also develop in women who engage in extreme exercise regimens. In these cases, restoring weight to a normal level and, if necessary, reducing the amount of exercise is often sufficient to restore fertility. Once weight has been normalized, fertility drugs may be recommended. The drug of choice is clomiphene, an antiestrogen drug that indirectly stimulates the ovaries to produce eggs. Medications to induce ovulation are effective in most women. If this treatment is not successful, the ovary can be directly stimulated by injecting either gonadotropins or gonadotropin-releasing hormones. Some disorders of the pituitary gland lead to excess production of the hormone prolactin, which can suppress ovulation. High levels of prolactin can be reduced by drugs such

# SITES OF FEMALE INFERTILITY

In women, infertility may be caused by abnormalities at a number of sites along the reproductive tract, including the ovaries, the fallopian tubes, the uterus, and the cervix. Problems sometimes are caused by a previous infection, an anatomic abnormality, or the results of an operation.

## Disorders of the fallopian tubes

Damage to the fallopian tubes sometimes results from certain infections, surgery on the pelvic organs, endometriosis, and sterilization. An ectopic pregnancy (one that develops outside the uterus) most commonly occurs in a fallopian tube. The surgery needed to treat this complication may permanently damage the affected tube.

## Disorders of the ovaries

In some women, infertility is caused by anovulation – the inability of the ovaries to produce mature eggs. Several conditions may cause anovulation, including excessive weight loss, obesity, ovarian failure, hormonal imbalances, or polycystic ovarian disease (an uncommon condition in which cysts develop in the ovaries). Permanent or temporary anovulation may also follow a severe illness or may occur suddenly for no identifiable reason.

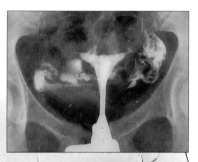

### Investigating ovarian disorders
*Ultrasound scanning, which monitors the growth and rupture of ovarian follicles, can provide evidence that ovulation is taking place. A sample of cervical mucus, taken at the time of ovulation, provides similar information. Spread on a slide and dried, it crystallizes in a typical fern pattern (below). Your blood can be examined to monitor your progesterone levels, which rise only after ovulation. Low levels of this hormone suggest that ovulation has not occurred.*

### Investigating fallopian tube disorders
*Hysterosalpingography is a diagnostic technique that introduces dye through the cervix, into the uterus, and finally through the fallopian tubes, where its progress can be monitored with X-rays (left). Laparoscopy is a more invasive procedure performed while the patient is under general anesthesia. The gynecologist passes a viewing instrument directly into the abdomen and watches dye moving into the pelvis. Laparoscopy is also used for diagnosis and treatment of other conditions such as endometriosis or adhesions (scar tissue as a consequence of surgery or infection).*

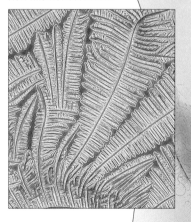

**Fallopian tube**   **Ovary**

**Uterus**

**Cervix**

## Disorders of the uterus

In rare cases, infertility can be caused by disorders of the uterus. For example, the uterus may be misshapen as a result of a congenital abnormality, or scar tissue can block all or part of the uterine cavity. Fibroids are a fairly common uterine disorder, but they are an uncommon cause of infertility. They lead to infertility only when they distort the cavity of the uterus to such an extent that they interfere with implantation of an embryo.

## Disorders of the cervix

The surface of the cervix is covered by cells that secrete mucus. Under the influence of ovarian hormones, this mucus becomes receptive to sperm at the time of ovulation and can act as a reservoir for them. Rarely, a woman's cervical mucus produces antibodies to her partner's sperm, causing infertility.

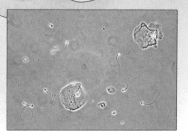

### Investigating cervical disorders
*Cervical mucus is usually examined in a postcoital test. The woman comes to her doctor's office within a few hours of intercourse and a sample of mucus is taken and examined microscopically.*

as bromocriptine, which inhibits the secretion of prolactin. Hypothyroidism, which is an uncommon cause of anovulation, may be treated with thyroid hormone; ovulatory function usually resumes within a few months.

## Other infertility treatments

For some infertile couples, conventional treatments are not successful and in vitro fertilization is the only way to achieve a pregnancy. Gamete intrafallopian transfer (GIFT) is a technique similar to in vitro fertilization and is less complex. Collected eggs are injected into the ends of the woman's fallopian tubes with the man's sperm. Fertilization can occur in its natural environment, the fallopian tube. GIFT can be used only in women with normal fallopian tubes. Zygote intrafallopian transfer (ZIFT) places an ovum fertilized in a laboratory into the woman's fallopian tube.

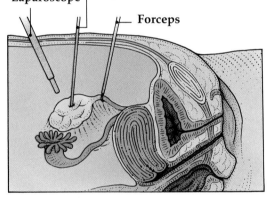

**Laparoscope** — **Aspiration needle**

**Forceps**

**Obtaining an egg**
*In the technique of gamete intrafallopian transfer, egg production is stimulated with fertility drugs. The eggs are collected by using an aspiration needle and a laparoscope.*

## MALE INFERTILITY

About 30 percent of all fertility problems are related to factors affecting the male partner. Several tests are used to investigate male infertility. The semen is always examined microscopically. Causes of male infertility include undescended testicles, blocked vasa deferentia (the

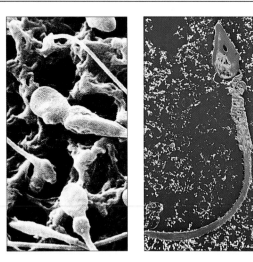

**Problems with sperm**
*All men produce semen with some dead or misshapen sperm (far left and left). In some men, the proportion of faulty sperm is high enough to reduce fertility. Other problems include sperm that cannot swim, and the production, by some men, of antibodies against their own sperm, causing the sperm to stick to each other.*

tubes that connect the testes to the urethra), and abnormal sperm. Problems with erection and premature ejaculation may be psychological in origin (in which case psychosexual counseling may help) or may be the result of diseased nerves or blood vessels in the genital area. Apart from surgery to correct some conditions, there are few treatments for male fertility problems. Self-help measures include improving general health by eating a nutritious diet, cutting down on alcohol and cigarettes, and reducing stress.

## UNEXPLAINED INFERTILITY

If a couple has regular, unprotected intercourse for 3 years without achieving a pregnancy and tests fail to reveal any fertility problems in either partner, treatment must progress without knowledge of the cause. Treatments include fertility drugs or introduction of semen directly into the uterus. The woman can be artificially inseminated with her partner's semen or, if he has a very low sperm count, the couple may decide to use a donor's semen. Artificial insemination is usually done along with ovarian stimulation to increase the number of follicles and therefore the number of eggs produced. For some individuals, in vitro fertilization, GIFT, or ZIFT results in a pregnancy when other treatment methods have failed.

---

**BLOOD TESTS**

Blood tests are occasionally helpful in establishing the causes of male infertility. Chromosome analysis is routinely carried out. The most common problem is an extra sex chromosome, a condition that cannot be treated. Hormone analysis provides information on the levels of hormones that stimulate the function of the testicles (gonadotropin hormones). High hormone levels suggest that the testicles have failed and sperm production has stopped. This condition is untreatable. Low hormone levels suggest that sexual development is incomplete. Antibody measurements detect excess production of spermatazoal antibodies. In such cases, treatment is possible.

# CASE HISTORY
# AN INABILITY TO CONCEIVE

S USAN AND BOB MARRIED **2 years ago and planned to start a family immediately. They have not been using any form of contraception. They have become concerned that Susan has not yet conceived. Furthermore, she has been experiencing pelvic pain for the last few months, particularly during her menstrual periods. Worried that the two problems may be linked, Susan decided to consult her gynecologist.**

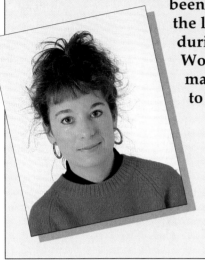

### PERSONAL DETAILS
**Name** Susan Porter
**Age** 28
**Occupation** Teacher
**Family** Susan's parents are both well and there is no history of disease in her family.

### THE CONSULTATION
The gynecologist explains that it is common for couples not to have achieved pregnancy after 2 years. He performs a pelvic examination to investigate the cause of Susan's pain. The gynecologist can feel that Susan's fallopian tubes are thickened and he decides that a laparoscopic examination is necessary.

### THE DIAGNOSIS
The laparoscopy confirms that Susan has ENDOMETRIOSIS, a disease not clearly understood, in which fragments of tissue resembling the endometrium (the lining of the uterus) grow outside of the uterus in other areas of the pelvis. In Susan's case, the condition has caused scarring and distortion of her fallopian tubes. Eggs produced by the ovaries and sperm are unable to move through the fallopian tubes, and fertilization cannot occur. The doctor asks Susan to bring her husband to the next appointment so that his fertility can be assessed as well.

Semen analysis evaluates the motility, viability, and shape of Bob's sperm, as well as the volume and consistency of his semen. The results show that Bob's semen is normal.

### THE TREATMENT
The gynecologist prescribes danazol, a synthetic hormone that opposes the effects of estrogen and causes endometrial tissue to wither. Because this treatment is not always successful, the doctor asks Susan to return in 6 weeks.

**Ultrasound scanning**
*During days 9 through 13, after taking the fertility drugs, Susan undergoes a series of ultrasound scans to monitor the ripening of the eggs in her ovaries.*

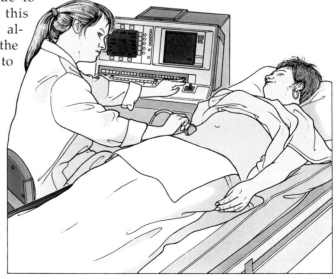

### FURTHER TREATMENT
At her next visit, Susan says that her pelvic pain has subsided, but another laparoscopic examination shows that danazol has not affected her scarred fallopian tubes. It is unlikely that treatment with a synthetic hormone will accomplish much more. The gynecologist tells Susan that, although her tubes are damaged, she has a normal uterus and she is a good candidate for in vitro fertilization. Susan takes fertility drugs to stimulate egg production. With the help of ultrasound, ripe eggs are removed from Susan's ovary just before ovulation and mixed with her husband's sperm in a dish that is then placed in an incubator. After about 40 hours, the gynecologist finds that fertilization has occurred and embryos are developing successfully. He passes them through Susan's cervix into her uterus.

### THE OUTCOME
Susan is observed for 5 days to determine that an embryo has safely implanted in the uterine wall. Once implantation occurs, her pregnancy continues. Later tests confirm that a fetus is developing normally.

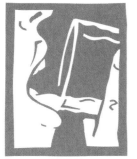

# URINARY TRACT PROBLEMS

URINARY TRACT PROBLEMS are common in women and can occur at any age. The symptoms produced may severely affect your quality of life but treatment is available. You can take steps to reduce the risk of urinary tract infections by drinking plenty of fluids and promptly obeying the urge to empty your bladder.

The urinary tract includes the two kidneys, two ureters (the tubes connecting the kidneys to the bladder), the urinary bladder, and the urethra (the tube connecting the bladder to the outside of the body). Common urinary problems that women experience include several types of cystitis and incontinence.

## BACTERIAL CYSTITIS

Bacterial cystitis is easy to recognize. It usually appears quite suddenly, often after sexual intercourse, and causes some or all of the following symptoms:

◆ Stinging and burning pain during urination
◆ The urge to urinate frequently, even when your bladder is empty
◆ Offensive-smelling urine
◆ Cloudy urine
◆ Blood-stained urine
◆ Pain in the lower part of your abdomen and back
◆ Fever

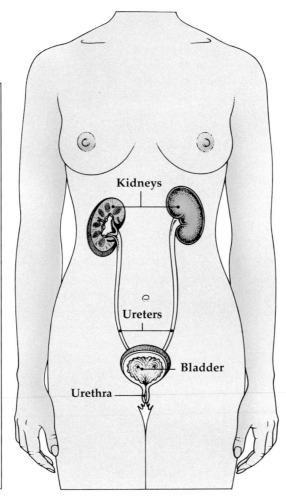

Kidneys

Ureters

Bladder

Urethra

## CYSTITIS

Cystitis describes any inflammation of the bladder, usually caused by infection or sometimes by chemicals such as some anticancer drugs. Most women experience cystitis at one time or another because it is relatively easy for infectious agents to pass from your urethral opening up into your bladder.

### Bacterial cystitis

The most common type of cystitis, which affects 10 to 20 percent of all women, is caused by bacterial infection of the bladder and urethra. The reason bacterial cystitis is so common in women – far more common than in men – lies in the anatomy of the female urinary tract. A woman's urethra is only 1 to 2 inches long (compared with about 10 inches in a man) and leads straight from the bladder to the outside, opening just in front of the vaginal entrance, an area where various bacteria are always present. Bacteria do not have to travel far to enter the bladder. In addition, because a woman's urethra lies next to her vagina, bacteria are easily massaged up the urethra during sexual intercourse.

**The urinary tract**
*The kidneys filter waste products from the blood and excrete them in the form of urine. The urine passes down the two ureters to be stored in the bladder until the bladder is full. The bladder then empties almost completely through the urethra, which opens just in front of the vagina.*

## TREATING BACTERIAL CYSTITIS

If you have an attack of cystitis, there are a number of ways you can help yourself get over it quickly and with as little discomfort as possible.

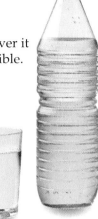

### Fluid intake
*Drinking plenty of fluids helps to flush the bacteria out of your bladder. Drink a pint of water initially, followed by half a pint every half hour. The burning that you feel when you urinate will gradually settle as the bacteria are washed away.*

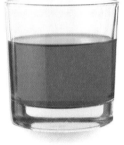

### Urine acidity
*Increasing the acidity of your urine helps relieve the burning sensation and pain caused by your bladder infection, as well as slow bacterial growth. You may be able to increase urinary acidity by drinking large quantities of cranberry juice. However, such a home remedy should not preclude consulting your doctor.*

### Medical advice
*If you suspect that you have a urinary tract infection, consult your doctor. He or she will ask you to provide a urine sample and will probably prescribe an antibacterial. You may also be advised to take a mild painkiller to reduce the pain and inflammation.*

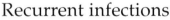

### PYELONEPHRITIS

A bacterial infection in the bladder can spread upward into the kidneys, leading to pyelonephritis (a kidney infection). This type of ascending infection is common in pregnant women. Pyelonephritis is a serious condition that may cause scarring of the kidneys and, ultimately, kidney failure. Treatment includes taking antibiotics and painkillers and drinking large amounts of fluids. You may even need to be admitted to the hospital.

## Recurrent infections

If you have a recurrent urinary tract infection, you may have a urethral, bladder, ureteral, or kidney abnormality that interferes with urinary flow. Your doctor can arrange for an ultrasound scan, a kidney X-ray, and cystoscopy (a procedure that enables your doctor to look inside your bladder with a viewing instrument). If no abnormality is found and you have cystitis only after sexual intercourse, your doctor may suggest that you take antibiotics before or after intercourse. This measure may be recommended for women who have more than four episodes of cystitis a year.

## ASK YOUR DOCTOR
## URINARY PROBLEMS

**Q** **I have had bacterial cystitis several times. I am now pregnant; is it true that a bladder infection can lead to miscarriage?**

**A** No. However, during pregnancy you are at increased risk of urinary tract infection. Consult your doctor at once if you have an attack of cystitis.

**Q** **My doctor says I have overflow incontinence and that I need to have more tests and be treated immediately. I have heard that pelvic floor exercises can help with incontinence. Should I try these exercises first?**

**A** No. Overflow incontinence occurs when the bladder does not empty correctly. It may be due to an underactive bladder or to obstruction of the urethra. Treatment should be carried out promptly, because the female bladder can stop contracting normally after being severely overdistended by retention of urine. Pelvic floor exercises are appropriate for and will help women with stress incontinence.

**Q** **Occasionally, I leak a little urine. I have had tests and my doctor tells me I am not suffering from incontinence. What could be the cause of my problem?**

**A** Abnormal bladder contractions can be provoked by certain situations such as hearing the sound of running water or putting the key into the lock of your front door. The contractions can bring on a sudden urge to urinate and may even cause slight leakage, particularly if you have been suppressing the need to empty your bladder.

## Interstitial cystitis

Interstitial cystitis, which is far less common than bacterial cystitis, is the term used to describe a long-standing inflammation of the space between the lining and muscle of the bladder. The exact cause of the condition is unclear, but it may result from bacterial infection or a reaction of the immune system. The symptoms of interstitial cystitis – bladder pain and a frequent, urgent need to urinate – may persist for many years. Antibiotics do not relieve the symptoms and the urine usually does not contain bacteria. Treatment is difficult.

Interstitial cystitis may cause ulceration of the bladder. Eventually, the bladder may become small and scarred; its capacity may be severely reduced. If you have severe, persistent interstitial cystitis, your doctor may suggest several types of surgery, including total removal of your bladder, enlargement of your bladder with a piece of your bowel, or stretching your urethra and bladder. Surgery is not always successful, and some operations have a higher success rate than others. Discuss the surgical options very carefully with your doctor and seek a second opinion.

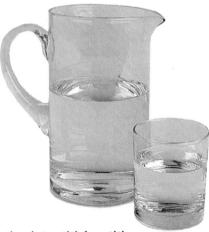

**Treating interstitial cystitis**
*Make sure you drink plenty of fluids (at least 2 quarts a day) to dilute your urine and make it less irritating to the inflamed bladder lining. Emotional stress can make the symptoms of interstitial cystitis worse and some women find psychotherapy can help relieve the condition. Some urologists instill medication directly into the bladder.*

## PREVENTING CYSTITIS

If you have had more than one attack of cystitis, there are a number of actions you can take to avoid infections in the future.

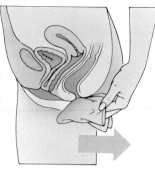

**Personal hygiene**
*Keep your genital area clean by washing morning and night. Make sure that you thoroughly rinse off soap. Do not use strong disinfectants because they may aggravate the problem. When you wipe yourself after a bowel movement, make sure you wipe from front to back to avoid contaminating your vulval area with fecal bacteria.*

**Clothing**
*Wear cotton underwear and loose-fitting clothes. Tight garments and underwear made of nylon or other synthetic fabrics keep the vulval area warm and moist, which promotes bacterial growth.*

**Tampons or pads**
*There is no conclusive evidence that tampon use causes urinary tract infections. You can use the type of sanitary protection you prefer – just remember to change tampons and pads regularly.*

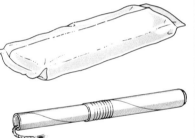

**Vaginal deodorants**
*Avoid the use of vaginal deodorants because these can irritate the vagina, vulva, and urethra and make them more susceptible to an attack of cystitis.*

**Sexual intercourse**
*It is not possible to prevent bacteria from entering the urethra and bladder during sex, so it is important to flush them out by urinating before and soon after sexual intercourse.*

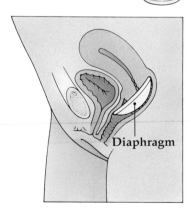

Diaphragm

**Contraceptives**
*Studies show that use of a contraceptive diaphragm significantly increases the risk of cystitis in some women. A diaphragm tends to compress your urethra, thereby reducing your urine stream and increasing the chance of bacteria being trapped within your bladder overnight. If you use a diaphragm and have recurrent urinary tract infections, you may want to ask your doctor about different methods of contraception.*

# CASE HISTORY
# PAINFUL URINATION

A FEW DAYS AFTER RETURNING from a vacation with her boyfriend, Michelle developed a burning pain every time she urinated. In addition, she felt an ache above her pubic bone and needed to pass urine more frequently than usual. Michelle had never experienced these symptoms before, and she immediately made an appointment with her doctor.

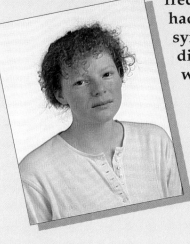

**PERSONAL DETAILS**
**Name** Michelle Davies
**Age** 24
**Occupation** Research scientist
**Family** Both parents are well. She has no children.

## MEDICAL BACKGROUND

Michelle had the usual childhood diseases, but has never had any major illnesses. She has no previous history of urinary tract problems, and has never contracted a sexually transmitted disease. Her periods have always been regular, and she takes a combined oral contraceptive.

## THE CONSULTATION

The doctor listens to Michelle's description of her symptoms. She then takes Michelle's blood pressure and examines her abdomen. The doctor discovers that Michelle is slightly tender in the lower part of her abdomen over her bladder. She asks Michelle to provide a urine sample and explains how to collect a sample that is uncontaminated by the contents of her genital tract. The sample is sent to the laboratory for culture and analysis.

## THE DIAGNOSIS

The doctor says that Michelle's symptoms are probably due to an attack of URETHROCYSTITIS caused by bacterial infection. She explains that bacteria present in Michelle's own body, particularly the bowel, may have been introduced into her urethra by the mechanical action of foreplay or sexual intercourse.

## THE TREATMENT

The doctor prescribes a course of antibacterial medication and advises Michelle to drink plenty of fluids. She explains that passing urine immediately before intercourse, and shortly afterward, can help prevent recurrence by flushing out as many bacteria as possible. She also tells Michelle that careful personal hygiene is very important, especially wiping from front to back after using the toilet and bathing regularly. The doctor reassures Michelle that her symptoms should disappear quickly. If the symptoms persist, the doctor tells her to return to the office in a few days for further treatment.

## THE OUTCOME

As predicted, Michelle's symptoms quickly disappear. When she calls the doctor's office, she is told that the laboratory results confirm a bacterial urinary tract infection. The doctor tells Michelle that the combination of self-help measures and antibacterial drugs has been successful in clearing up the infection. Michelle is relieved to discover that she does not have a serious disorder, and that an attack of this type of urethrocystitis is a common problem.

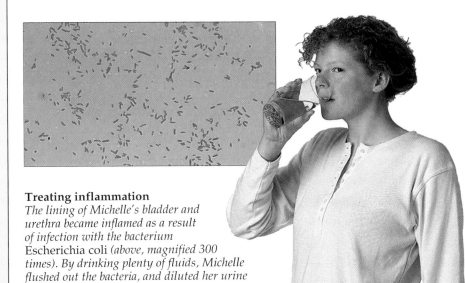

**Treating inflammation**
*The lining of Michelle's bladder and urethra became inflamed as a result of infection with the bacterium* Escherichia coli *(above, magnified 300 times). By drinking plenty of fluids, Michelle flushed out the bacteria, and diluted her urine to make it less irritating to the inflamed tissue.*

# COPING WITH INCONTINENCE

Urinary incontinence is the term for the involuntary loss of urine. It is most common in older women. However, as many as 40 percent of women between 30 and 50 also experience it. Although it is natural to feel embarrassed about this type of problem, do not postpone seeking medical help. In most cases, treatment can improve or even completely cure incontinence. There are many causes of involuntary loss of urine, but the two most common are stress incontinence and urge incontinence, which together account for more than 90 percent of the cases.

**Bladder control**
*Normally, the bladder fills and empties without any change in its internal pressure – more like a plastic bag than a balloon. When the bladder is full, it signals to the brain that it is ready to contract and expel urine. Usually, the brain suppresses this reflex until it is convenient for you to empty your bladder. When you are ready, your brain stops suppressing the urge, the bladder muscle is allowed to contract, and the muscles of the pelvic floor and urethral sphincter relax, allowing urine to pass down the urethra.*

## HOW IS THE BLADDER CONTROLLED?

**The bladder and urethra**
*The bladder is a hollow muscular organ that stores urine and then releases it down the urethra. The bladder muscle (detrusor muscle) is joined to the muscle of the urethra, but the urethra also has a band of circular muscle fibers around it known as the urethral sphincter. This sphincter muscle (together with the muscles of the pelvic floor) retains urine in the bladder until you voluntarily relax it.*

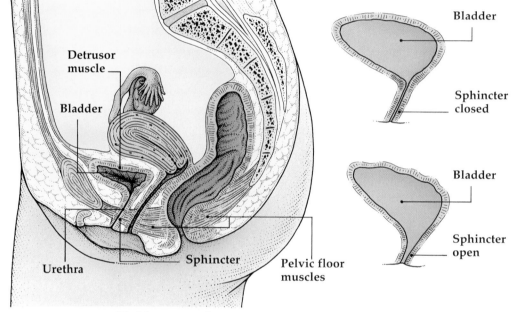

Detrusor muscle

Bladder

Urethra

Sphincter

Pelvic floor muscles

Bladder

Sphincter closed

Bladder

Sphincter open

## URGE INCONTINENCE

Sudden uncontrolled loss of urine is known as urge incontinence, detrusor instability, or bladder instability. Usually, no obvious reason can be found for it but doctors believe that it may occur in women who did not learn bladder control as children. Sometimes the condition is due to a neurological disorder such as stroke or multiple sclerosis.

**Bladder contractions**

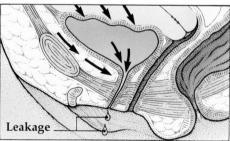

Leakage

**Why urge incontinence occurs**
*Urge incontinence occurs when the normal suppression of bladder function by the brain is absent and the bladder contracts at inappropriate times. Drug therapy may be prescribed to inhibit the bladder contractions. Some women with severe urge incontinence may need surgery to correct the problem.*

**Gaining bladder control**
*To regain bladder control, reeducate your bladder to urinate by the clock rather than by the urge. Start by emptying your bladder every half hour to an hour during waking hours and do not urinate in between, even if this results in leakage. Once you are on this schedule, increase the interval by half an hour until you can control bladder function.*

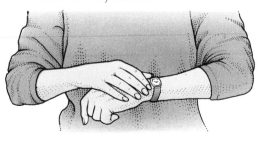

## STRESS INCONTINENCE

Stress incontinence is caused by incompetence of the urethral sphincter. It can also occur as a result of weak pelvic floor muscles. These muscles are particularly likely to be stretched during pregnancy and childbirth or may also be weakened by a chronic cough and constipation. Increasing age and the menopause may also lead to stress incontinence. Treatment for stress incontinence is usually surgery, which has a 70 to 95 percent success rate.

**Why stress incontinence occurs**
*Stress incontinence occurs when the pressure within your bladder is raised without an equal rise in pressure in your urethra. Coughing, sneezing, or lifting a heavy weight often causes increased intra-abdominal pressure on your bladder.*

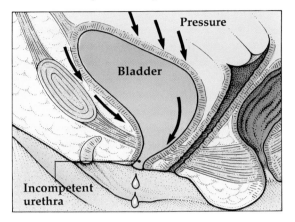

Pressure

Bladder

Incompetent urethra

### PELVIC FLOOR EXERCISES

The most popular alternative to surgery for genuine stress incontinence is the practice of pelvic floor muscle exercises. These exercises are designed to improve the strength and tone of your pelvic floor muscles. Exercise cures stress incontinence in about 25 percent of cases and improves symptoms in another 25 percent. Younger, premenopausal women who have less severe symptoms and who may be motivated to perform the exercises are most likely to benefit. This form of treatment does not require hospitalization or time off work and does not have any side effects.

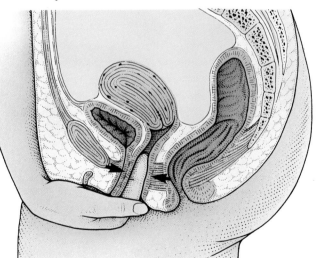

**1** First try to identify your pelvic floor muscles by using them while you urinate to interrupt your flow. Another method of locating the muscles is to place two fingers in your vagina and try using the muscles to squeeze the fingers (right).

**2** Once you can feel your pelvic floor muscles, deliberately contract them at regular intervals throughout the day (but not while you are urinating). It is best to hold each contraction for about 5 to 10 seconds and to perform the exercise 50 times per day. You will probably begin to notice a stronger response from the muscles within 3 or 4 weeks.

**Vaginal cones**
*Some doctors recommend training pelvic floor muscles with a set of cone-shaped vaginal weights (right). Successively heavier cones are inserted into the vagina until the heaviest cone can be held in place for 15 minutes. Many women are unwilling to use them.*

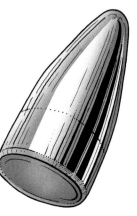

**SELF-HELP FOR INCONTINENCE**

Limit your fluid intake to 3 pints a day. Ask your doctor to make sure that you do not have a urinary tract infection. If you are taking diuretic drugs, ask him or her to reevaluate your treatment. If you have passed the menopause, you may benefit from hormone replacement therapy. If you leak only while exercising vigorously, you may find that wearing a tampon during exercise reduces the leakage. If nighttime frequency is a problem, try not to drink anything in the evening and urinate before going to bed. Cut down on drinks that have a diuretic effect such as tea, coffee, and alcohol. If incontinence remains a problem, ask your doctor or pharmacist for appropriate pads and pants to minimize your discomfort.

# BREAST DISORDERS

**M**OST WOMEN CONSIDER their breasts an important part of their female identity and are concerned about any change in the character of one or both breasts. All women need to be aware of disorders that can affect the breasts and able to recognize warning signs of these disorders at an early, treatable stage.

Breasts differ widely in size, shape, and texture from one woman to another. The shape, size, and color of the nipples also vary. It is normal for a woman to have one breast that is larger than the other. However, any sudden change in the character of your breasts should be checked by your doctor. The appearance of a lump in the breast is always frightening. However, most breast lumps are benign (noncancerous) and 50 percent of women have benign breast lumps at some time in their lives.

## MAMMOGRAPHY

Mammography is a simple procedure in which an X-ray is taken of each breast. Breast cancers usually contain tiny calcium deposits, which can be detected on the X-ray film long before they can be felt. One study showed that deaths from breast cancer could be reduced by 30 percent with regular use of mammography. Every woman should have a mammogram once between 35 and 40 years of age, every 1 to 2 years between 40 and 50, and annually after age 50.

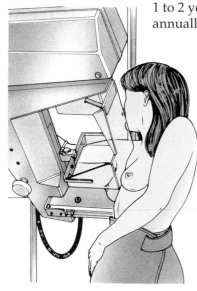

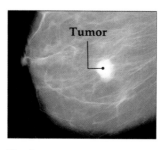

Tumor

**Having a mammogram**
*Your breast is placed on a machine and compressed between the X-ray plate below and a plastic cover above. The irregular, dense mass in the mammogram above represents a tumor.*

## INVESTIGATING BREAST CHANGES

All women should know how to examine their breasts and should take the time to do so regularly (see WHEN SHOULD I CONSULT MY DOCTOR? on page 78). If you find any changes in your breasts, see your doctor as soon as possible. You probably have a noncancerous condition. But if cancer is present, early diagnosis is vital because cancer is more effectively treated in its early stages.

### Biopsy
If you or your doctor finds a lump in your breast, it must be evaluated. This may involve examination of your breast by your doctor, mammography, aspiration of the lump with a needle, and/or biopsy. The intensity of the investigation and the number of tests performed are determined by the doctor's judgment of the likelihood of malignancy.

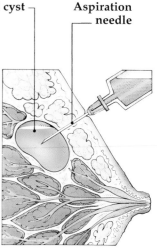

Fluid-filled cyst

Aspiration needle

**Needle aspiration**
*Needle aspiration (fine needle biopsy) of either cystic (fluid-filled) or solid masses may be performed. Cells obtained from solid masses and from the fluid in cystic masses are examined under a microscope. A lump that persists after aspiration should be removed and examined for signs of malignancy.*

# SURGERY OF THE BREAST

Removal of all or part of the breast is called mastectomy and is usually performed to treat breast cancer (see page 123). The type of operation done and the amount of the breast removed depend on the size and location of the tumor, the extent to which the cancer has spread, and the age and health of the woman. Most doctors explain that the option of minimal surgery, while less disfiguring, carries a small risk of recurrence of the cancer. Postoperative checkups are essential. The doctor also may prescribe anticancer drugs and radiation therapy to increase the chances that all cancer cells are destroyed. Reconstructive surgery and the use of implants can help restore the appearance of the breast.

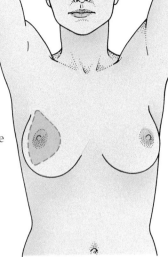

**Lumpectomy**
A lump in the breast is removed along with a layer of surrounding tissues. Healing leaves a barely noticeable scar. The procedure has cured many women with breast cancer without the need for a mastectomy. Radiation treatment is also usually used to reduce the risk of recurrence.

**Partial mastectomy**
The tumor is removed along with the overlying skin, a portion of the surrounding tissues, and some of the underlying tissues. Radiation treatments are usually required.

**Subcutaneous mastectomy**
Only the internal breast tissue is removed, leaving the nipple and skin intact. A silicone implant usually replaces the breast tissue that has been removed. This procedure is not done to remove cancer. It has been used to prevent cancer in women at high risk.

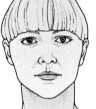

**Simple mastectomy**
The entire breast is removed, but the pectoral (chest wall) muscles and the lymph nodes in the armpit are preserved.

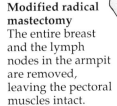

**Modified radical mastectomy**
The entire breast and the lymph nodes in the armpit are removed, leaving the pectoral muscles intact.

**Radical mastectomy**
The breast, lymph nodes in the armpit, and pectoral muscles are all removed. This disfiguring operation, which is no more effective than a simple or modified radical mastectomy, is almost never performed today.

# BREAST PROBLEMS

Cancer is not the most common disorder affecting the breast. At least 80 percent of breast lumps found by self-examination (such as those described here) are benign and are caused by disorders other than cancer. However, for women, breast cancer is the second major cause of death from cancer, after lung cancer. Although the incidence of breast cancer is increasing for reasons that are not fully understood, early detection and advances in treatment have kept the death rate stable over the past 50 years.

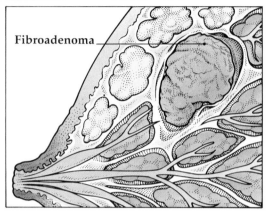

**Fibroadenomas**
*Fibroadenomas (above) are benign, fibrous growths in the breast. They can grow at any stage of a woman's fertile years from the onset of menstruation to the menopause. However, they are most common in women under 30. Fibroadenomas are distinct, painless lumps that are very mobile because they are not attached to any structure in the breast.*

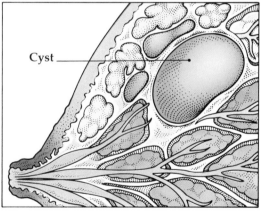

**Breast cysts**
*Breast cysts (above) may result from obstruction of a milk duct. Usually the blockage is caused by fibrosis (an overgrowth of scar or connective tissue). However, cysts are sometimes caused by cancer. The cysts contain clear yellow or blue-green fluid and are treated by needle aspiration. The extracted fluid is examined under a microscope to ensure that no cancerous cells are present.*

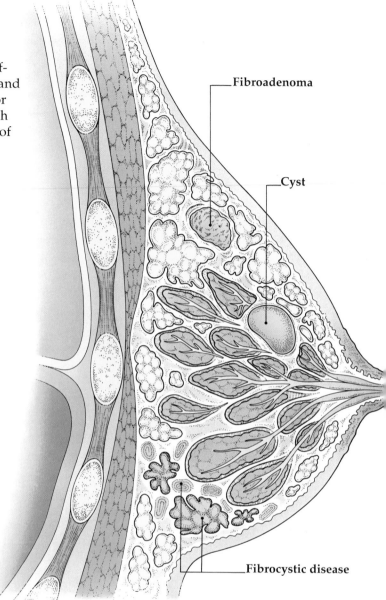

**Fibrocystic breast disease**
*Fibrocystic breast disease (right) is characterized by an increase in the fibrous and glandular tissue in the breast. This increase sometimes results in the formation of cysts. The condition usually causes pain and a feeling of lumpiness in the breast toward the end of a menstrual cycle. Mammography may be performed to rule out cancer. There is no specific treatment for fibrocystic disease. However, diuretic drugs may relieve the tenderness in the breasts. If symptoms are severe, the hormone progesterone or the drug danazol may be prescribed.*

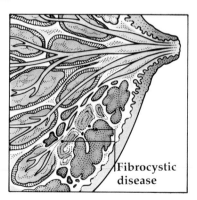

# BREAST CANCER

Breast cancer will develop at some time in approximately one in every nine women. Sixty percent of malignant tumors (below right) are found in the upper, outer quadrant of the breast, and they often spread via the lymphatic system (which explains the importance of checking the lymph glands in your armpit during self-examination).

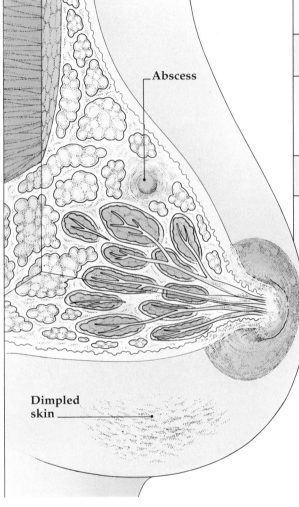

Abscess

Dimpled skin

| LESS COMMON BREAST DISORDERS | |
|---|---|
| **Papilloma of the milk duct** | A benign tumor that grows in a milk duct (the ducts that carry secretions from the tissues of the breast to the nipple). The first symptom is usually a bloody discharge from the nipple. |
| **Mammary duct ectasia** | A widening of a milk duct. This rare condition usually affects postmenopausal women. |
| **Fat necrosis** | A condition usually resulting from injury in which fat cells of the breast die, leaving tough scar tissue that may form a firm or calcified nodule visible on a mammogram. |
| **Galactocele** | A cyst containing milk that sometimes occurs after pregnancy. |
| **Paget's disease of the nipple** | A rare, malignant condition in which a tumor grows in the openings of the milk ducts in the nipple. The condition looks like eczema and causes the nipple to itch and burn. It occurs mainly in postmenopausal women. |
| **Sarcoma** | A very rare type of malignant breast tumor that grows from tissues supporting the breast tissue. |
| **Galactorrhea** | A spontaneous and persistent production of milk by a woman who is not pregnant or breast-feeding. The condition is sometimes caused by medications or, uncommonly, by an excess secretion of the hormone prolactin as a result of dysfunction or a tumor of the pituitary gland. |

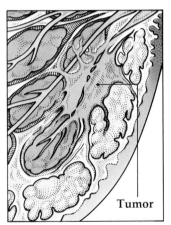

Tumor

**Symptoms of breast cancer**
*Apart from a lump in the breast, which is the most common warning sign of breast cancer, other symptoms and signs include swelling, tenderness, discharge from the nipple (far left), indentation of the nipple, and a dimpled appearance of the skin overlying a lump (left). In more than 90 percent of cases, only one breast is affected.*

**Breast abscess**
*A breast abscess (below) is a collection of pus in the breast tissue caused by infection. Abscesses are most common in breast-feeding women because bacteria tend to enter the breast through a cracked nipple. An abscess may cause tenderness and, if it is close to the skin, inflammation. Antibiotics are prescribed to treat the infection, and the abscess may be drained of pus.*

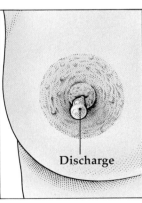

Discharge

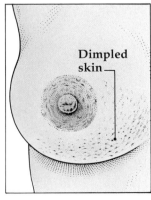

Dimpled skin

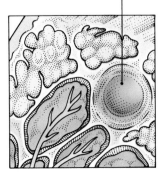

Abscess

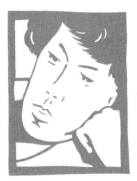

# MENOPAUSAL PROBLEMS

**M**ANY WOMEN GO THROUGH the menopause without any problems. However, if you have symptoms that may be caused by the menopause, talk to your doctor. Treatment can help relieve your symptoms. Your doctor may also want to make sure the symptoms are not caused by some other condition.

**Vaginal changes**
*As your level of estrogen decreases, the cells that make up the lining of your vagina shrink (atrophy). Cells from the lining of a premenopausal vagina and cells from the lining of a vagina with atrophy are shown at right, (magnified 160 times). The vagina itself becomes drier, less acidic, and more susceptible to infection.*

With the onset of the menopause, a woman's ovaries stop functioning and she produces decreasing amounts of estrogen. As a result, some immediate and some long-term changes take place.

## CHARACTERISTICS OF THE MENOPAUSE

During the years leading up to the menopause, a woman's menstrual periods usually become shorter, lighter, and less frequent, although they may become heavier or more frequent.

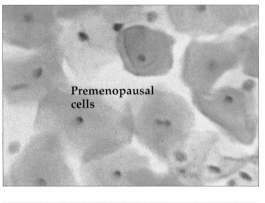

Premenopausal cells

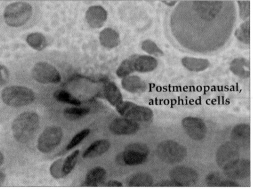

Postmenopausal, atrophied cells

Periods may not occur for several months, then recur irregularly until they stop altogether. They may stop suddenly and completely. Some women find that their premenstrual symptoms become worse as the menopause approaches.

## Vaginal dryness and atrophy

Vaginal dryness is a relatively common problem in postmenopausal women. As the estrogen level decreases, the reproductive organs – including the uterus, vagina, and vulva – gradually shrink (atrophy). The inner lining of the vagina may become dry and thin. These changes can cause genital irritation, burning, and itching. Sexual intercourse may be uncomfortable or painful and may cause bleeding. Use of a lubricant in and around the vagina before penetration makes intercourse more comfortable for many women. Estrogen tablets, creams, or suppositories can prevent or reverse vaginal dryness and atrophy.

## Urinary problems

Lack of estrogen also affects the tissues of the urinary tract; thinning and wasting can increase the risk of infection. Symptoms include burning pain during urination, sudden urges to urinate, increased urinary frequency, and loss of bladder control (incontinence). The symptoms often improve with hormone replacement therapy (see page 34) or with other drugs if hormone replacement therapy is not recommended.

## Sexual problems

A decrease in sexual interest and desire is sometimes a menopausal problem. It is often a result of the pain or discomfort during intercourse caused by vaginal atrophy. It can also be caused by hormonal and emotional changes. A woman's sexual life need not be affected by the menopause. Hormone replacement therapy can resolve the problems caused by vaginal dryness and can often restore sexual desire if it has diminished. Evidence suggests that regular sexual intercourse helps maintain sexual responsiveness and enjoyment. Sexual relations can be more enjoyable after menopause because pregnancy is no longer a concern. Partners also may be more experienced and more relaxed with each other at this stage of their lives.

## Psychological problems

Some menopausal women suffer from fatigue, memory loss, irritability, anxiety, or depression. These problems are usually not permanent or serious. They are sometimes accompanied by the sleep disturbance that results from night sweats. Hormonal changes and emotional factors may play a part. Psychological problems at this time of life should not simply be attributed to the menopause. Concern about aging and uncertainty about the future are common causes of emotional problems during the menopause. Other causes of stress, such as problems at work or within the family, may also be important factors. Don't deny your emotional difficulties. Talking about them with a friend or relative – or a counselor – often helps.

**EARLY MENOPAUSE**

A woman who goes through the menopause early (before 40) is at increased risk of osteoporosis and heart disease due to long-term estrogen deficiency. If the ovaries are removed before the menopause, estrogen deficiency symptoms may appear within days of the operation. Hormone replacement therapy is almost always recommended for such women.

## HOT FLASHES AND NIGHT SWEATS

About 75 percent of women experience hot flashes during the menopause. When hot flashes occur at night, they are called night sweats (see HOW DO I RECOGNIZE THE MENOPAUSE? on page 32). These conditions can usually be treated effectively by hormone replacement therapy. Hot flashes are sometimes prevented with clonidine, a drug that is also used to treat high blood pressure, if hormone replacement therapy cannot be used.

As described here, hot flashes occur with a surge of a hormone produced by the pituitary gland. Yet women who have undergone removal of the pituitary gland still have hot flashes. Clearly, the underlying cause is not fully understood.

**Pituitary gland**

**2** This pituitary hormone alters the regulation of blood vessel size and body temperature.

**Coping with hot flashes**
*Hot flashes can be aggravated by stress, spicy foods, alcohol, tea, and coffee, so you may benefit from avoiding these items. Certain drugs that are usually used to treat endometriosis may also cause hot flashes. Your clothing can affect the intensity of a hot flash; dress in easily removable layers and avoid wearing heavy clothing that fits tightly around your neck.*

**1** Hot flashes are probably triggered in the hypothalamus (a region of the brain). Hormonal secretions may cause a surge of a hormone produced by the pituitary gland.

**3** Body temperature rises and blood vessels dilate, causing hot flashes and night sweats.

**4** Hot flashes may be accompanied by sweating and redness of the skin.

# TAKING CARE OF YOURSELF DURING MENOPAUSE

One positive way to approach the menopause is to take good care of yourself. Women who are healthy, fit, and emotionally well adjusted are the least likely to experience major problems around the time of the menopause or in later years. Don't smoke or drink too much alcohol. Make it a point to eat balanced meals, exercise regularly, and avoid excessive stress. If you have problems or concerns, discussing them with a sympathetic listener can help you bring their importance into perspective. Professional caregivers such as doctors and counselors can offer you reassurance, explanations, and practical recommendations, as well as advice on treatment with hormone replacement therapy or other drug therapies to relieve symptoms.

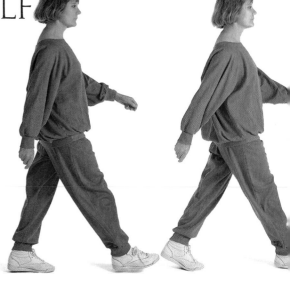

### Diet
*A balanced diet is vital to good health. An inadequate intake of some nutrients may increase the risk of diseases associated with aging. Make sure you get enough vitamins, minerals, and essential fatty acids by eating a varied diet that includes a wide selection of fruits, vegetables, nuts, whole-grain breads, protein, and dairy products.*

### Visiting a clinic
*There may be a women's health clinic in your area with staff members who are trained to work with women who have menopausal problems. At these clinics, medical personnel offer health education, discuss concerns, perform medical examinations, and prescribe treatment.*

### Exercise
*Exercising regularly helps increase the density and strength of your bones and slows down the rate of loss of bone tissue. Exercise is of much greater value if you start well before the menopause. The amount of exercise you get should be equivalent to walking at least 1 mile each day.*

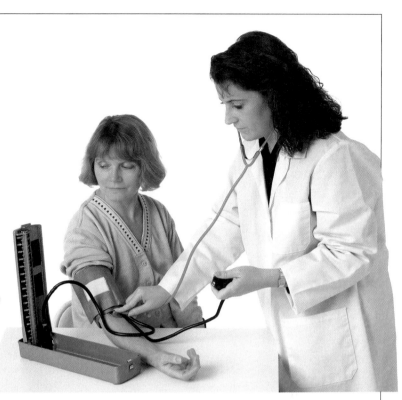

### Talking it over
*Talk about your symptoms, problems, or feelings with friends who are going through the same experiences. You may find it reassuring to learn that other women are having similar physical and emotional experiences.*

### Regular medical checkups
*Regular medical checkups are important at any time of life. They should include blood-pressure checks, breast and pelvic examinations, and urine tests. Cancer of the cervix is still common after the menopause, so it is important that you continue to have regular cervical (Pap) smears.*

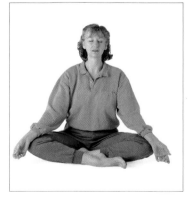

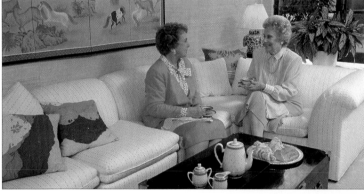

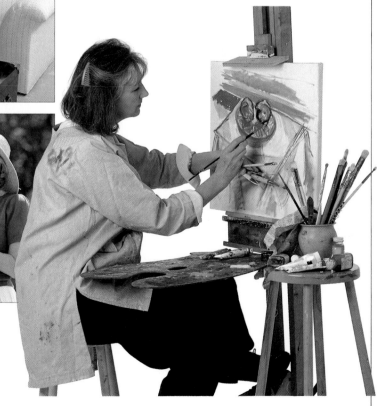

### Learning to relax
*If you can relax and cope with stress, you will be better equipped to cope with any menopausal symptoms. You may find it helpful to do relaxation exercises to relieve tension. Hobbies and social activities can help introduce periods of pleasure and calm into your daily life.*

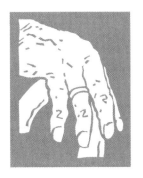

# PROBLEMS OF THE OLDER WOMAN

L ETHARGY, LOSS OF APPETITE, confusion, falling, and immobility are problems that should never be regarded as unavoidable consequences of the aging process. Such symptoms indicate that you have some disorder. In many cases, the disorder is treatable. Talk to your doctor about any persistent health problem.

In a young person, the appearance of any symptom is usually immediately noticeable. As we grow older, it is easy to become accustomed to intermittent, sometimes subtly progressive symptoms. You should not ignore these symptoms because they may be treatable and they may be signs of the onset of disease.

## CANCER

The fear of cancer is a common concern among older Americans. However, if the disease is detected early enough, treatment is often successful. Seek medical attention promptly if any of the following warning signs develop:

◆ Persistent cough
◆ Lump in your breast or elsewhere
◆ Change in bowel habits
◆ Unusual bleeding or discharge
◆ Change in a wart or mole
◆ Sore that does not heal
◆ Change in bladder habits
◆ Persistent indigestion
◆ Difficulty swallowing
◆ Persistent hoarseness

**Cardiovascular disease**
*As we get older, our cardio-vascular system deteriorates and blood pressure often begins to rise. Disorders in the system can cause chest pain (angina), breathlessness, dizziness, and confusion. Severe cardiovascular disease may result in heart failure, myocardial infarction (heart attack), or stroke.*

**Arteries harden,** lose elasticity, and become narrowed by fatty deposits (atherosclerosis).

## HEALTH DISORDERS OF LATER LIFE

As you grow older, it is particularly important to pay close attention to the signals you receive from your body. You should report to your doctor any change for which there is no explanation.

### Fractures

After the menopause, women become more likely to fall and more likely to suffer fractures, particularly of the spine, hip, and wrist, because their bones become weakened by osteoporosis (see page 130). Compression fractures of the vertebrae are painful and temporarily disabling. Hip fractures can be particularly serious. Between 10 and 15 percent of older women who fracture a hip die as a result; many others are left severely disabled. The keys to avoiding post-menopausal fractures are preventing osteoporosis and preventing falls (see AVOIDING FALLS on page 133).

**Heart valves** become calcified.

**Heart valve**

**The efficiency** of the heart declines.

## Genital bleeding

Any loss of blood from the genital tract after the menopause is called post-menopausal bleeding. If you are having hormone replacement therapy with estrogen and a progestin, you can expect monthly bleeding. Whether or not you are having hormone replacement therapy, you should report any other blood loss to your doctor.

Postmenopausal bleeding has a variety of possible causes, including cancers of the endometrium (lining of the uterus), cervix, vagina, or vulva. Other causes are vaginal dryness, polyps of the cervix or uterus, and hyperplasia (excessive growth) of the endometrium. Bleeding may also occur as a result of damage to thinned and wasted vaginal tissues during sexual intercourse. If you are undergoing hormone replacement therapy, another possibility is that your hormone dosage may need adjustment.

## Depression

Some older adults experience episodes of depression. Older people may encounter both financial and psychological difficulty adjusting to retirement. Feelings of loneliness and isolation are common, particularly among women and men who have lost their partners. Illness, disability, and loss of independence may also contribute to depression. Signs that a person may be depressed include apathy, sleeping difficulties, loss of appetite, and self-neglect. Other characteristics of depression are overwhelming feelings of hopelessness, worthlessness, and guilt. Depression is not an inevitable consequence of aging. Do not hesitate to seek help from your doctor if feelings of depression are interfering with your enjoyment of life.

## Dementia

The term dementia describes a general impairment of intellect, memory, and personality. About 2 percent of people between 65 and 75 suffer from dementia.

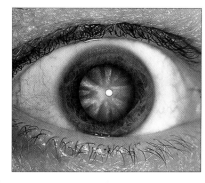
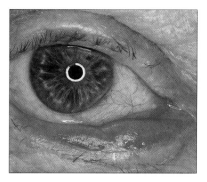

**Eye problems**
*By age 65, nine out of 10 people have farsightedness (difficulty focusing on near objects). This condition, also called presbyopia, can easily be corrected with glasses. Many other eye problems also become more common with increasing age, including glaucoma, which is increased pressure in the eye; cataracts (above left); ectropion, which is outward turning of the eyelids (above right); and entropion, which is inward turning of the eyelids.*

The figure rises to more than 15 percent in people over 80. About 55 percent of dementia cases are caused by Alzheimer's disease, which is a progressive disorder of the brain. The precise cause of Alzheimer's disease remains unknown but is currently the subject of research. Dementia may also result from other conditions – commonly from disturbance of blood supply to the brain (from multiple small strokes) or from vitamin $B_{12}$ deficiency or thyroid underactivity.

## Other problems

A variety of other health problems become more common in older women. Talk to your doctor if any worrisome symptoms last for more than a few days.

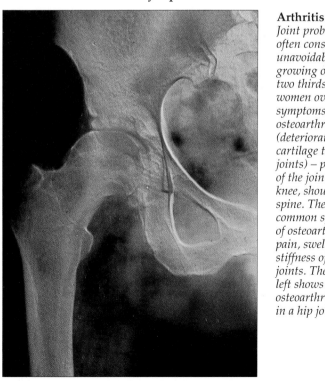

**Arthritis**
*Joint problems are often considered an unavoidable part of growing old. About two thirds of all women over 65 have symptoms of osteoarthritis (deterioration of the cartilage that lines joints) – particularly of the joints in the hip, knee, shoulder, and spine. The most common symptoms of osteoarthritis are pain, swelling, and stiffness of the affected joints. The X-ray at left shows osteoarthritic changes in a hip joint.*

# WHAT IS OSTEOPOROSIS?

Osteoporosis is a common condition in which the density of your bones decreases. Your bones become thin, brittle, and increasingly vulnerable to fractures. Osteoporosis is a major health problem; it affects one out of every four women and leads to more than 1.5 million fractures each year in the US. In addition to causing distress and disability, the complications of many of these fractures – particularly those of the hip – are fatal to older victims.

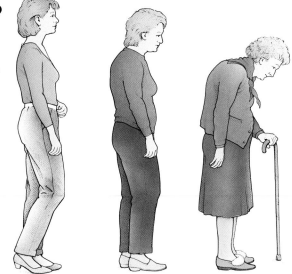

**Age 35 and over    Age 65 and over    Age 75 and over**

## EFFECTS OF OSTEOPOROSIS

Osteoporosis develops gradually over many years. The bones become progressively thinner without any change in their shape. Health problems tend to begin when about 30 percent of bone mass is lost. A bone may be broken by the stress of a minor accident or your spine may start to compress and cause back pain.

**Spinal changes**
*Osteoporosis causes the bones in the spine to weaken and become less able to support the weight of the upper part of the body. The bones can become compressed, resulting in loss of height and spinal curvature and causing a stooped posture that becomes more pronounced with age (above).*

### WHO IS AT RISK?

Although bone density naturally decreases with age, some women are more susceptible than others to osteoporosis. Important risk factors are:

◆ Early menopause
◆ Genetic factors (women of European and Asian descent are more at risk than those of African descent)
◆ Low calcium intake
◆ Cigarette smoking
◆ Excessive alcohol consumption
◆ Being underweight
◆ Anorexia nervosa
◆ Childlessness
◆ Immobility and lack of exercise
◆ Long-term corticosteroid therapy (often prescribed for asthma, inflammatory bowel disease, or severe skin diseases)

**Fractures**
*Fractures of the wrist and neck of the femur (top of the thighbone) are typical and immediately apparent. An X-ray showing a fracture of the neck of the femur is shown at far right. Fracture of one or more spinal vertebrae are less obvious – but often very painful – because affected bones are compressed rather than snapped.*

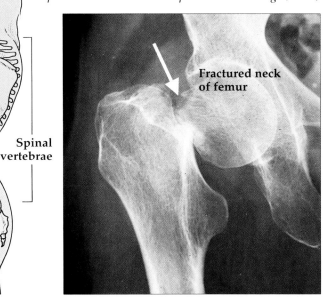

**Spinal vertebrae**

**Wrist**

**Neck of femur**

**Fractured neck of femur**

**Loss of bone tissue**
*Your bone is a living substance consisting of tissue that is continually being broken down and replaced by new tissue. However, as you get older, the amount of tissue being broken down can exceed the amount of tissue being replaced. Over time, the bones become less dense and more brittle. This is an effect of aging; bone mass is gradually lost from the skeleton from about age 35 onward. The rate of bone loss speeds up considerably when your estrogen level falls during and after the menopause.*

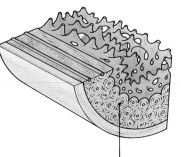

**Normal, dense bone**

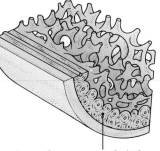

**Less dense, more brittle, osteoporotic bone**

**Preventing osteoporosis**
*The most effective weapon against osteoporosis is prevention – ideally starting in childhood. Regular exercise and plenty of sunshine help build strong bones that are less likely to become osteoporotic (see* REDUCING THE RISK OF OSTEOPOROSIS *on page 44). In addition, your diet should include plenty of calcium-rich foods such as low-fat dairy products, green leafy vegetables, whole grains, and beans (right).*

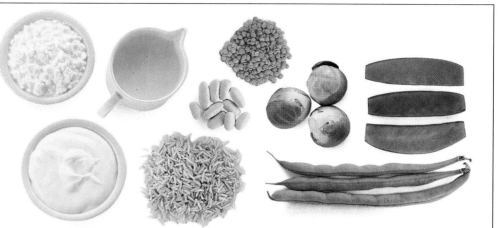

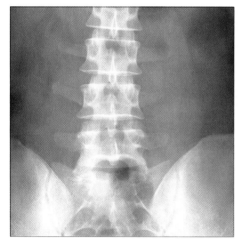

**Diagnosing osteoporosis**
*Osteoporosis can be diagnosed using X-rays. The X-ray above shows a normal spine; the X-ray below shows osteoporotic changes of the vertebrae. Dual photon densitometry, a technique that measures bone density by exposing the bone to a harmless source of radioactivity and recording the amount of radiation absorbed, is being investigated. Blood and urine tests are also used to rule out other bone diseases such as those caused by overactivity of the parathyroid glands.*

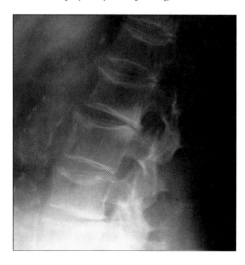

## DRUGS FOR OSTEOPOROSIS

The use of drugs to prevent and treat osteoporosis is a subject of much medical research and debate. The drugs described in this chart may be given alone or in combination.

| Drug | Advantages | Disadvantages |
| --- | --- | --- |
| **Hormone replacement therapy** (see HORMONE REPLACEMENT THERAPY on page 34) | Increases calcium absorption, limits bone loss, and reduces the incidence of fractures if taken for at least 5 years starting at menopause. | Cannot effectively restore bone tissue, so is of limited benefit if osteoporosis is already established. Also causes some monthly bleeding. |
| **Calcitonin** (a hormone produced by the thyroid gland) | Regulates the way bones absorb calcium from the blood, can help prevent bone loss, and can reduce the risk of fracture. | Cannot be taken orally but has been developed as a nasal spray. Causes side effects such as nausea, vomiting, and flushing and tingling of the hands. |
| **Etidronate** One of a group of drugs called diphosphonates, which are primarily used to treat Paget's disease, a bone disorder; its use for the treatment of osteoporosis is investigational. | May decrease bone loss, increase bone density, and reduce the incidence of fractures. May be more effective than hormone replacement therapy or calcitonin in increasing bone density. | Causes side effects such as nausea, diarrhea, and increased bone pain. |
| **Calcium supplements** Widely used, although their exact value is not established. | Strengthen bones. | Play only a minor role in preventing bone loss. |
| **Fluoride supplements** | Can stimulate bone formation and increase bone density. | Any bone formed may be abnormal and as likely to fracture as osteoporotic bone. |
| **Vitamin D** | Helps increase the amount of calcium in bone and may help reduce the rate of vertebral fractures. | Can raise the amount of calcium in the blood to abnormally high, even dangerous, levels. |

# TAKING STEPS TOWARD HEALTH

We cannot stay forever young, but we can take positive steps to preserve our health and mobility. Quitting smoking is essential in preventing the premature aging of the skin, lungs, bones, and heart that the addiction can cause. Staying active reduces your dependence on other people. Pursuing your interests challenges your mind and provides stimulating contact with other people.

## Taking medication

Many older people need medications and they often must take several drugs at the same time. It is difficult to follow a complicated drug schedule and to remember to take each dose at the right time. You may find some of the following suggestions helpful, particularly if you are taking drugs over a long period of time.

Write down instructions as your doctor gives them to you. You may wish to make a list on a calendar of the drugs you have to take each day and check off each dose as you take it. No matter how good your memory is, it is always a good idea to keep a written record of the drugs you are taking and their correct dosages. Make sure that all your drug containers are clearly labeled with their contents and directions. Dispose of any surplus drugs and any drugs that have passed their expiration date by flushing them down the toilet.

## AIDS FOR THE DISABLED

Many types of equipment, including glasses, hearing aids, walkers, and wheelchairs (and other mobility aids), are available to enable impaired or disabled people to function more easily. In addition, there are many devices specially designed to reduce the difficulty of everyday household tasks such as washing, cooking, and cleaning.

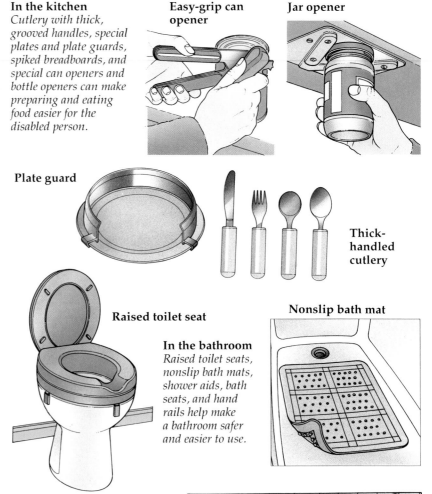

**In the kitchen**
*Cutlery with thick, grooved handles, special plates and plate guards, spiked breadboards, and special can openers and bottle openers can make preparing and eating food easier for the disabled person.*

**Easy-grip can opener**

**Jar opener**

**Plate guard**

**Thick-handled cutlery**

**Raised toilet seat**

**In the bathroom**
*Raised toilet seats, nonslip bath mats, shower aids, bath seats, and hand rails help make a bathroom safer and easier to use.*

**Nonslip bath mat**

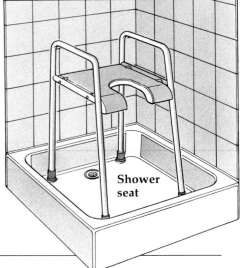

**Shower seat**

**Aids to taking medications**
*If you are using several medications and find it difficult to keep a record of the time at which each one has to be taken, try using a special multiple-medication box (right). These boxes contain compartments, labeled with the days of the week and times of the day, into which you can place your daily quota of medications. If you have been prescribed tablets that are difficult to swallow, ask your doctor whether your drug is available in liquid form.*

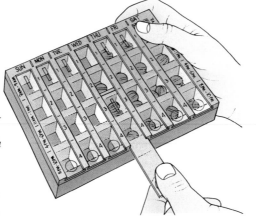

**Dressing aids**
*Long-handled shoehorns, dressing sticks, elastic shoelaces, front-fastening bras, and attachments to zipper pulls can all make dressing easier.*

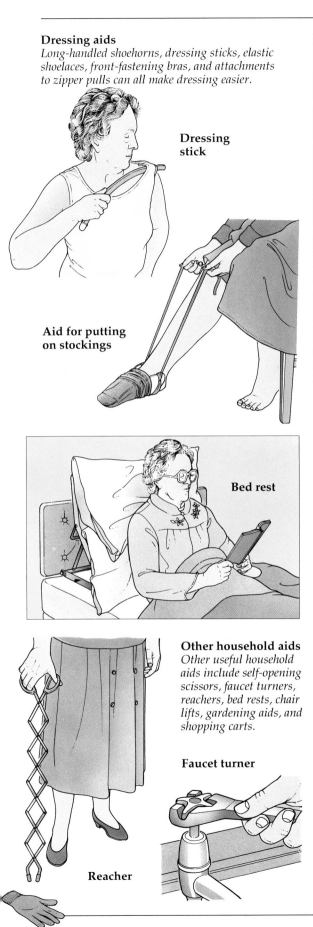

**Dressing stick**

**Aid for putting on stockings**

**Bed rest**

**Other household aids**
*Other useful household aids include self-opening scissors, faucet turners, reachers, bed rests, chair lifts, gardening aids, and shopping carts.*

**Faucet turner**

**Reacher**

# AVOIDING FALLS

Accidental falls are common among women over 65. Each year, about one third of all older people accidentally fall in their homes, sometimes with serious consequences. Falls can result in cuts, fractures, head injuries, and burns, as well as loss of confidence. In some cases, a fall can be fatal. You can help guard against falls by taking precautions every time you go outside your home. You can also make adjustments in your home to make it safer.

◆ Use a cane or a walker if you're unsteady on your feet.

◆ Choose well-fitting footwear; if your shoes have shoelaces, make sure they are tied securely.

◆ Wear glasses if you need them, but take off reading glasses before moving around.

◆ Secure any loose electrical wiring.

◆ Make sure carpet edges are well anchored.

◆ Try to ensure that floors are not slippery.

◆ Do not place loose rugs on slippery floors.

◆ Install handrails near the bath and toilet.

◆ Use nonslip mats in and alongside the bath or shower.

◆ Ensure that all stairways have strong banisters.

◆ Keep a lamp or flashlight by your bedside.

◆ Make sure that lighting is adequate, particularly over stairs and in other potentially hazardous places.

◆ Store frequently used items in easily accessible places so that you do not have to climb to reach them.

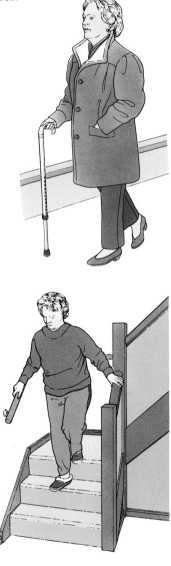

**Why do people fall?**
*Falls occur because agility and balance naturally decrease with age. In addition, falls are a common complication of disorders such as poor vision, joint problems, or muscle weakness.*

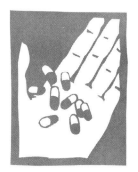

# ANXIETY AND DEPRESSION

ANXIETY AND DEPRESSION are common problems. Rapid social change and an increasingly complex society create conflict and stress for many of us. About 9 million Americans have depressive disorders, and it is estimated that one woman in four will experience serious depression at some time in her life.

Evidence suggests that the tendency to become anxious or depressed is a trait that runs in families. Relatives of people who suffer from anxiety are five times more likely to become anxious than the general population, and relatives of people who experience depression are 10 times more likely to become depressed. However, extremely severe stress is usually necessary to turn a genetic susceptibility for anxiety or depression into an anxious or depressive state. Stressful life events, including the death of a partner or relative, divorce, illness, and job concerns, increase the risk of anxiety or depression. Paradoxically, events that are regarded as happy, such as getting married or having a baby, can have similar temporary effects. If you are depressed or anxious, talk about your symptoms with your family doctor.

## ANXIETY

Feelings of anxiety can be beneficial, alerting you to a need to take action to resolve a threat. Anxiety for which treatment may be required is a fear reaction that is characterized by sustained feelings of apprehension, sweating, rapid heart rate and breathing, excessive uneasiness, and a constant state of tension in the body. An effective way to prevent excessive anxiety is to minimize the number of major stresses that are occurring in your life at any one time. Try to plan ahead so that you do not change too many aspects of your life at once. If events pile up on you, it helps to talk over problems with someone else – a friend, member of the clergy, or counselor.

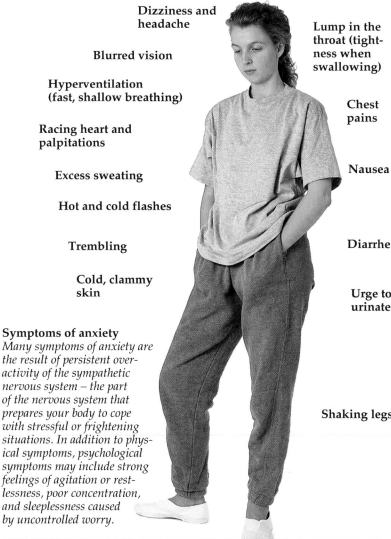

Dizziness and headache

Blurred vision

Hyperventilation (fast, shallow breathing)

Racing heart and palpitations

Excess sweating

Hot and cold flashes

Trembling

Cold, clammy skin

Lump in the throat (tightness when swallowing)

Chest pains

Nausea

Diarrhea

Urge to urinate

Shaking legs

**Symptoms of anxiety**
*Many symptoms of anxiety are the result of persistent over-activity of the sympathetic nervous system – the part of the nervous system that prepares your body to cope with stressful or frightening situations. In addition to physical symptoms, psychological symptoms may include strong feelings of agitation or restlessness, poor concentration, and sleeplessness caused by uncontrolled worry.*

## LEARNING HOW TO RELAX

Relaxation is an essential part of reducing the potential ill effects of stress. You may find relaxation in leisure pursuits, exercise, meditation, or massage. Alternatively, a tranquil state of mind may be achieved by practicing relaxation exercises in which you consciously tighten and relax each group of muscles in your body in a progressive sequence.

**Breathing**
*Do this breathing exercise before and after the other relaxation exercises. Take a slow, very deep breath; hold it to the count of 4. Breathe out very slowly to the count of 4. Repeat four times.*

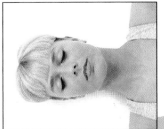

**Face**
*Close your eyes, slightly open your mouth, and raise your eyebrows. Then lower your brows to their resting position.*

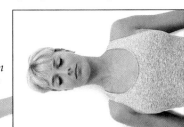

**Shoulders**
*Pull your shoulder blades together and down toward the floor; then flatten and spread them against the floor. Relax your muscles by returning to the original position.*

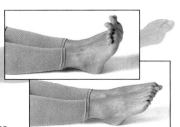

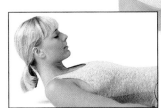

**Buttocks**
*Push your buttocks hard against the floor; hold for 4 seconds. Then relax.*

**Toes**
*Curl your toes downward for a count of 4. Then curl them toward your face for 4 seconds. Relax them.*

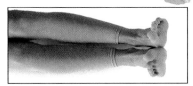

**Head and neck**
*Lower your chin to stretch the muscles in the back of your neck. Bend your head backward to stretch the muscles in the front. Bring your head back to its usual position.*

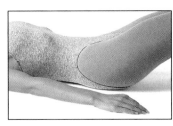

**Stomach**
*Tense your abdominal muscles by tightly holding them in for a count of 4. Relax them.*

**Calves**
*Point your feet toward your face by flexing your ankles and hold for a count of 4. Then relax.*

## Treating anxiety

If your anxiety persists or escalates, you may need professional counseling or individual psychotherapy. Supervised group discussions help some people become more confident and reduce the physical symptoms of their anxiety. Antianxiety medications can also reduce symptoms. Barbiturates and benzodiazepines are highly addictive and doctors are cautious about prescribing them. Beta blockers, which are drugs often used to treat high blood pressure, are also prescribed to reduce the rapid heartbeat and trembling associated with panic attacks. Beta blockers have other side effects but can be useful in the short term to control the symptoms of anxiety. Professional psychological support, along with relaxation techniques such as slow, deep breathing exercises, offers you more lasting benefits.

## Phobias, obsessions, and compulsions

Other forms of severe anxiety include phobias, obsessions, and compulsions. Phobias are fears of particular objects or situations that do not usually frighten most people. Phobias cause anxiety that can be reduced only by completely avoiding or leaving the cause of the fear.

**Common phobias**
*Agoraphobia (fear of open spaces or entering public places) and other phobias such as fear of thunderstorms (right) or heights (far right) affect women more than men. Social phobia (fear of social contact) is equally common among women and men.*

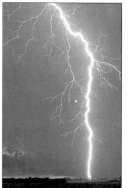

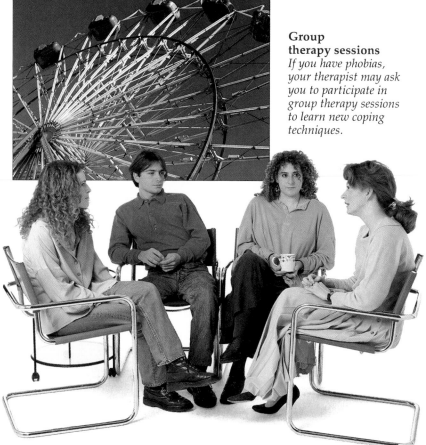

**Group therapy sessions**
*If you have phobias, your therapist may ask you to participate in group therapy sessions to learn new coping techniques.*

Obsessions are spontaneous, intrusive thoughts that cause anxiety and may lead to a compulsion - an urge to perform a repetitive, unnecessary act (such as washing hands that are already clean). Obsessive-compulsive behavior was once considered a rare problem, but about 3 percent of the US population is affected. People with phobias, obsessions, or compulsions are sometimes treated with behavior therapy. Others may be helped by medication or psychotherapy.

# DEPRESSION

Depression has many forms, but common features include profound sadness, pessimism, low self-esteem, inability to enjoy life, loss of energy, loss of interest in sex, loss of ambition, fatigue, headache, and insomnia. An attack of depression is sometimes signaled by a reduction in energy and loss of appetite. Severe depression may lead to loss of weight, constipation, and sleep disturbances – especially waking early in the morning. Many women and men feel depressed at some time in their lives, but rates of depression are twice as high for women as for men. While the causes of depression are still not fully understood, it is clear that genetic, biochemical, and environmental factors can all play a role.

## Suicide and attempted suicide

Women are more likely than men to attempt suicide and women are three times more likely to attempt suicide than to complete the act of suicide. Young women account for more than 60 percent of all hospital admissions for attempted suicide. Adolescent girls are four to five times more likely than boys to attempt suicide, but boys are much more likely than girls to die, mainly because boys choose more lethal methods. Some theories suggest that, because of the way women and men are trained, women feel more able to ask for help – even by attempting suicide.

**Women and depression**
*Studies show that women have higher rates of depression than men during both adolescence and adulthood. Hormonal fluctuations, such as those before menstruation and during pregnancy and childbirth, may provide a partial explanation for women's mood swings. Many other factors, related to life changes and a woman's willingness to acknowledge her depressed state of mind, probably also influence reported rates of depression.*

## Treatment for depression

Only one in 50 people with depression is admitted to the hospital, but many others need professional guidance to help them confront the cause of their disorder. Loving support from family and friends along with psychotherapy help the vast majority of depressed people recover. Antidepressant drugs are particularly useful to restore appetite and energy. For a person with severe, suicidal depression that has not responded to drugs, electroconvulsive therapy, in which an electric shock is passed through the brain for several seconds, can be effective. The physiological action of electroconvulsive therapy is not fully understood. In many cases, the treatment can result in dramatic improvement. However, it also may impair mental function to some degree.

**Postpartum depression**
*More than half of all new mothers experience some degree of depression within the first month after childbirth. Several factors may contribute to the "baby blues," including changes in hormone levels as a woman's body goes from a pregnant to a nonpregnant state, sleep deprivation, and emotional adjustments to motherhood. Very rarely, severe postpartum depression develops and requires psychiatric treatment.*

**Beating postpartum depression**
*Most women find that postpartum depression lifts without medication or therapy. If your feelings of depression persist or deepen, talk to your doctor.*

## ASK YOUR DOCTOR
## ANXIETY AND DEPRESSION

**Q** The last few times I have been to the grocery store, my heart has started to race and I have become dizzy. What is wrong with me?

**A** Your symptoms suggest a form of agoraphobia. Your body reacts as if you had to defend yourself or run away from some fear-inducing cause. This reaction causes a racing heart, rapid breathing, and shaking because oxygen-rich blood is being diverted to your limbs. Talk to your family doctor about your feelings and ask him or her if therapy would be appropriate in your case.

**Q** I have had difficulty sleeping lately. Although I go to bed early, I stay awake worrying about my problems. What can I do?

**A** Your insomnia may be the result of anxiety. Talk over your worries with a friend and take some steps to address your problems. If your symptoms persist, talk to your doctor. Exercise regularly, do not nap during the day, and do not drink tea or coffee toward the end of the day.

**Q** I am 50 years old and going through the menopause. For the last few months I have been very depressed. What can I do?

**A** Your feelings of depression may have little to do with the process of menopause. You may be experiencing some major changes at this time that are causing your depression. You may wish to turn to some form of career or retirement counseling or psychological therapy as you plan for your mature years. If physical symptoms of the menopause are troubling you, talk to your doctor.

# CARING FOR AN AGING RELATIVE

An older relative who becomes unable to take care of herself or himself can be a worrisome responsibility as the person becomes more dependent on you. Many women assume the role of primary caregiver when a spouse or other family member becomes ill or less able.

Many of the disorders common among older people, including psychological problems such as depression, can be treated effectively to improve the person's quality of life. Other conditions, such as congestive heart failure, require specialized care and a period of convalescence in a nursing home or at home. After recovery, it may be possible for the person to live at home either alone or with assistance from you, another relative or friend, or a professional caregiver.

**Diet and nutrition**
*Poor diet can be a cause of deteriorating health in older people who are unable to shop and prepare balanced meals. A diet of convenience foods may lack essential nutrients. You can help by shopping for the person or arranging for meal delivery.*

## ACTING ON A DOCTOR'S ADVICE

If a doctor thinks that your relative is unable to live alone, you need to decide whether you can take care of him or her or if you will need to arrange for long-term care. Your choice depends on how much care your relative requires and on how much time you can devote to him or her. Supportive family care is always beneficial, but not all family members have the resources to properly care for a disabled older person. Before you take on the responsibility of caregiving, gather as much information as possible about what you will need to do.

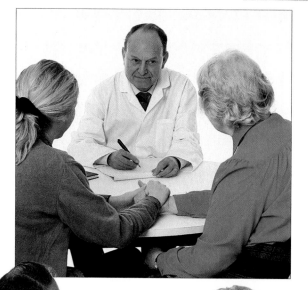

**A doctor's evaluation**
*The first step in making sure that you are providing the best care for an older, possibly disabled relative is to arrange for his or her doctor to make a medical evaluation of the person's condition. The form of care that is most satisfactory will depend on a number of factors, including the home environment and his or her health and ability to cope with everyday activities. The doctor will need to obtain a full medical, social, and psychological evaluation from you and your relative.*

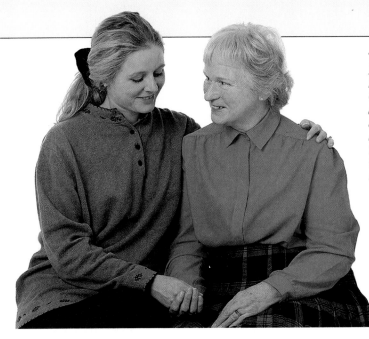

### The caregiving experience
*If your aging, impaired relative comes to live in your home, be prepared for considerable adjustments. Caregiving for an ill or disabled person can be demanding and exhausting, particularly if the person has dementia or other psychological conditions along with any physical difficulties. You will need patience and understanding if behavior becomes inappropriate. Encourage your relative to be as self-sufficient as possible and seek support from community resources if you need help.*

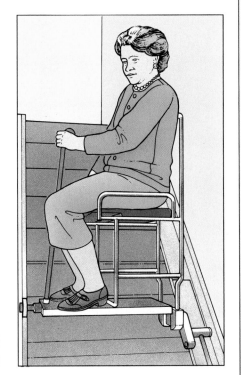

### Domestic aids
*Special aids around the house can be useful to an aging person who wishes to remain independent and live at home. Handrails can be invaluable to an arthritic or weakened person and are particularly useful in a bathtub or shower (right). Special elevators are available to help a person confined to a wheelchair move between floors (far right). Canes and walkers help with mobility. For those people who cannot leave the house or who cannot cook, a hot meal can be delivered daily through special arrangements.*

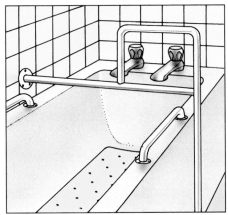

## CHOOSING A NURSING HOME

If you decide that you cannot provide your relative with the time or attention that he or she needs, you may decide to look for a nursing home. Try to locate a place that is easy to visit and not too far from your home. Arrange to meet the staff and residents before making a commitment, ask about state licensing requirements, and make sure that the home has proper facilities for your relative's needs. Ask the residents for their opinions of the home, and consider their comments in terms of the personality and needs of your loved one. Most homes for the aged are expensive. Make sure that you are fully aware of the long-term financial costs before committing yourself.

### Sharing interests
*When older people are no longer able to live in their own home, some prefer to live with people their own age rather than with their children because other older people have similar concerns and interests.*

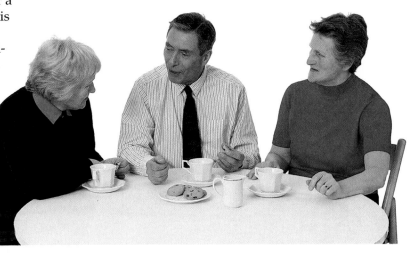

# VIOLENCE AGAINST WOMEN

Acts of violence against women range from verbal harassment to rape. Domestic violence is the most common cause of injuries to women in the US – 22 to 35 percent of women who visit emergency rooms have been abused at home. In recent years the number of reported rape cases has increased significantly. These chilling facts make it obvious that every woman needs to know how to protect herself against attack and what to do if she is attacked by someone she knows or by a stranger.

## A GUIDE TO SELF-PROTECTION

If you are assaulted or molested by a member of your family, seek help immediately because the attacker will almost certainly repeat the offense. Contact a women's crisis center, a shelter for battered women, or another counseling service, and leave home if you can. To help reduce the risk of attack by a stranger, take the precautions outlined below. Learning self-defense and assertive behavior can also help you prevent a crime against yourself. Rape is a crime of violence, not of sexual passion.

### AT HOME

◆ Install and use strong locks on all doors and windows.

◆ Install and use peepholes and safety chains on your outer doors and always see who is at your door before opening it.

◆ Put only your first initials and last name on your doorbell, mailbox, and in the phone book.

◆ Keep doorways and landings well lit.

◆ Get to know neighbors you can trust in case of an emergency.

◆ Do not open the door to any service person without checking his or her credentials; if you think it is necessary, telephone the employer for verification.

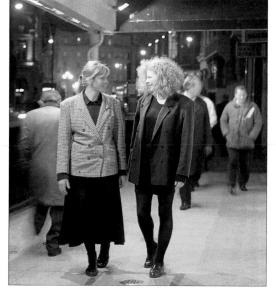

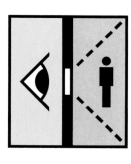

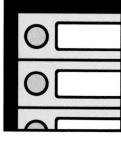

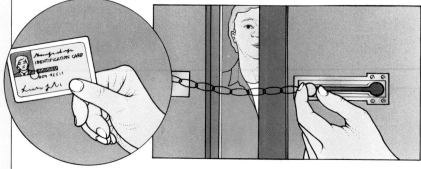

### ON THE STREET

◆ Walk with a companion at night; avoid run-down or abandoned buildings or poorly lit areas, and walk in the middle of the street in deserted areas.

◆ Always stay alert to what is happening around you and walk at a steady, determined pace to show that you know where you are going and to appear confident.

◆ Wear unrestrictive clothes and flat shoes so that you can move and run quickly.

◆ Carry a whistle or rape alarm in your hand; if you think that you are being followed, scream for help.

◆ If a driver stops to ask for directions at night, do not stop walking or get very close to the car.

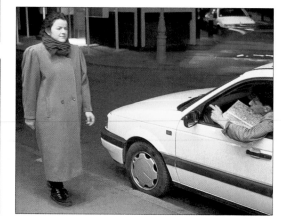

## TRAVEL

◆ Keep your car doors locked and windows shut while driving; always make sure that no one is hiding in your car before getting in.

◆ When on a bus or train, sit close to the driver or conductor, sit in an aisle seat near an exit, and stay awake at all times.

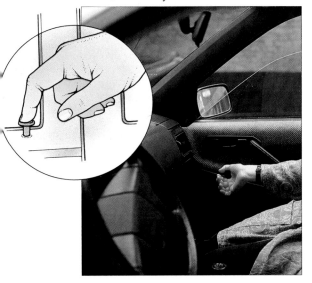

### Self-defense and assertiveness

*Although an attack is not the woman's fault, studies show that a woman who looks afraid is more likely to be harassed or assaulted. Training in self-defense enables you to better defend yourself and gives you a more confident air, which may help prevent attacks. Assertiveness training also can give you more self-assurance, which might discourage a would-be attacker. Many men will stop harassing a woman who forcefully tells them to "get lost."*

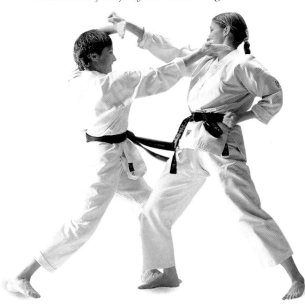

## WHAT TO DO IF YOU HAVE BEEN RAPED

If you have been raped or if you are with someone who has been raped, call the police immediately. Rape is a crime in every state. Next, call a relative, friend, or a rape hotline (or a community agency that offers rape counseling) to help you. Then call your doctor or the hospital emergency room to let them know that a rape has occurred and that you or another person will need medical treatment. The rape victim should not change clothes, shower or bathe, or brush her teeth. Physical effects of rape – which vary according to the nature of the attack – may include severe pain; bleeding; visible cuts, burns, and bruises; or unconsciousness. Profound anxiety, fear, and feelings of degradation are common.

**DO NOT allow the victim to:**

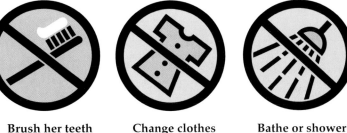

| Brush her teeth | Change clothes | Bathe or shower |

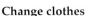

**Number of cases reported**

90,000
80,000
70,000
60,000
50,000
40,000

1970   1974   1978   1982   1986

**Year**

### Incidence of reported rape in the US

*The graph (left) shows a significant increase in the number of rapes reported annually in the US since 1970. It is not clear whether these figures reflect a genuine increase in the incidence of rape or a greater willingness on the part of victims to report the crime.*

### Reporting a rape

*Victims of rape are often reluctant to report the crime because they feel ashamed. Also, they may be concerned that the police and courts will be unsympathetic. It is estimated that a high percentage of rapes still go unreported. If you are raped, your report – difficult as it is to make – may be the only way to apprehend the rapist and save another woman from being* 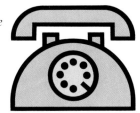 *similarly victimized. At the hospital, a policeman or policewoman, a rape counselor, and members of the medical staff may all be present to help. You will be asked to describe what happened several times, and a doctor will perform a physical examination to check you for sexually transmitted disease and to establish proof that the rape occurred.*

**Photograph sources:**
Ace Photo Agency **82** (bottom left)
Biophoto Associates **63**; **96** (top left); **112** (top left); **117**
Bridgeman Art Library **10** (top left); **59**
The Image Bank **9** (top right); **44** (center); **44** (bottom left); **49** (bottom right); **73**; **90** (bottom right); **107**; **126**; **127** (center)
Images Colour Library **46**
National Medical Slide Bank, UK **99** (bottom right); **130**
The Photographers Library **27**; **77**
Pictor International **2** (bottom left); **10** (top right); **30**; **49** (top right); **58** (top left); **85** (bottom center); **86**; **127** (bottom center); **136**
Picture Bank Photo Library **90** (center)
Saint Bartholomew's Hospital **97** (top right)
Saint Mary's Hospital **98** (top left)
Science Photo Library **2** (bottom right); **2** (top left); **11**; **15** (top left); **26**; **94** (bottom left); **96** (bottom right); **98** (bottom right

and left); **99** (top left and bottom left); **102**; **108**; **111** (top right); **112** (top right); **120** (center); **124**; **129** (top right); **129** (bottom center); **131**
Dr Albert Singer **102**
Tony Stone Worldwide **15** (bottom right); **49** (center); **141** (bottom left)
Telegraph Colour Library **9**; **45** (center); **48**
Andy Walker, Little Ashton Hospital **111** (bottom left); **111** (bottom right)
Dr Ian Williams **129** (top right)
James C. Webb **94** (top left)
Zefa **2** (top right); **7**; **10** (bottom right); **19** (bottom center); **36**; **41**; **44** (top center); **45** (top left); **45** (bottom left); **51** (bottom left); **55**; **76**; **85** (bottom right)

**Front cover photograph:** The Image Bank

**Index:** Sue Bosanko

**Illustrators:**
Russel Barnet
Joanna Cameron
Karen Cochrane
Peter Cox
David Fathers
Tony Graham
Andrew Green
Grundy & Northedge
Lydia Umney
Philip Wilson
John Woodcock

**Commissioned photography:**
Steve Bartholomew
Susannah Price
Clive Streeter

**Airbrushing:**
Paul Desmond
Roy Flooks

Reader's Digest Fund for the Blind is publisher of the Large-Type Edition of *Reader's Digest*. For subscription information about this magazine, please contact Reader's Digest Fund for the Blind, Inc., Dept. 250, Pleasantville, N.Y. 10570.